A Love Letter

By Wongel Gebeyehu

A Love Letter

By Wongel Gebeyehu © 2025

Published by Wongel Gebeyehu, Calgary, Canada.
ISBN: 978-1-0693286-1-8
Registered in Canada

Amharic Editor
Mekonnen Adamu

English Translator
Yonas Gezahegn

Cover And Layout Graphics
Girmachew Habtie Belay
+251 929377222

Publication assistance by

PAGEMASTER
PUBLISHING
PageMaster.ca

Notice

In my story, all the events recounted are genuine. However, I would like to inform my readers that I have changed the names of some individuals in certain instances, as I deemed it unnecessary to mention their real names.

Table of Contents

Chapter Four

Chapter Five

Chapter Six

Chapter Seven

Chapter Eight

Chapter Nine

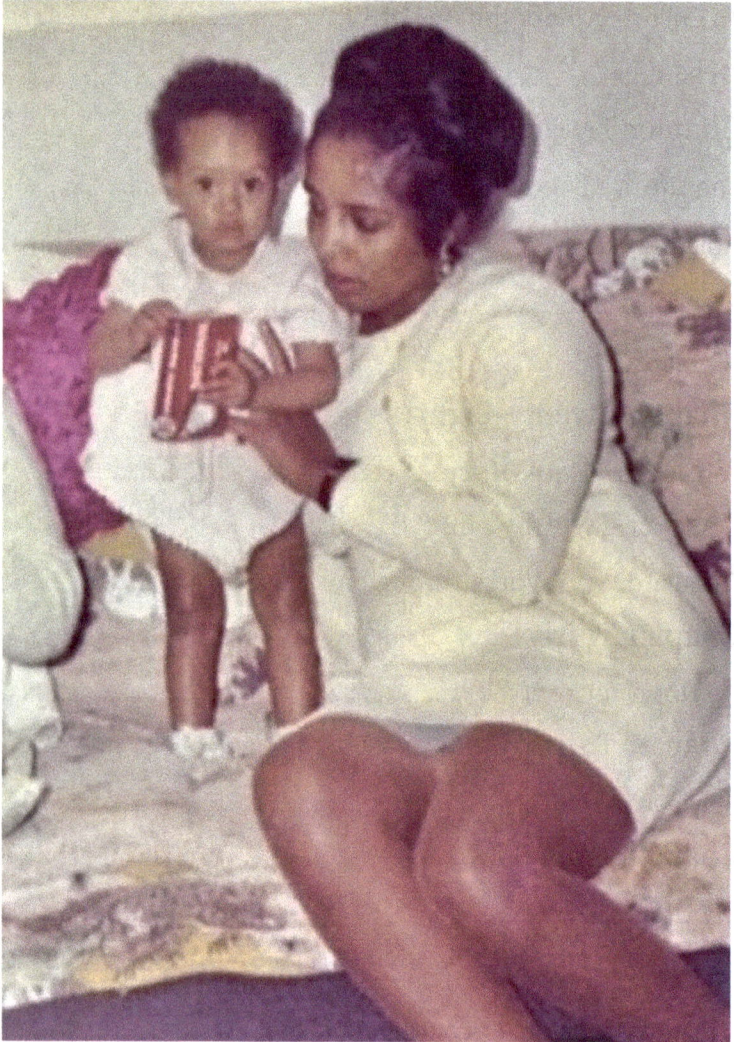

I want to dedicate this book to my dear mother, Mrs. Genet Fentaw who became my role model in every aspect of my life.

Dedication

This book is dedicated in memory of all individuals around the world who have been affected by cancer. Their courage and resilience are acknowledged here, and this work stands as a tribute to their strength and spirit.

Beta Readers' Comments

Our Sister **Wongel Gebeyehu** is widely recognized for her love and respect for others. She has been a significant blessing to our church community. Over the past ten years, despite facing her own challenges, she has consistently prioritized the needs of others and remained committed to fostering the love of Christ in the hearts of the young members of our congregation.

In her writing, she shares practical ideas that reflect the wisdom gained from her life experiences and many years of ministry, presented in a clear and accessible manner. Furthermore, she highlights the important issue of depression, which has been affecting our community recently, urging us not to overlook it. Thank you, Sister Wongel, for sharing this "Love Letter" with your readers.

Pastor Meron welde-Hawariyat
Pastor of Global Mission Faith Ministries calgary Canada

Wongel has been known to me for the past three decades. As a beta reader, I had the opportunity to review her manuscript. This book details God's faithfulness to Wongel as she faced the trials of being a cancer patient and throughout her life's journey. Wongel shares her keen observations on how we, as Christians, often react to fellow believers who are suffering from illness. She also provides guidance on what not to say or do in these situations. In this way, Wongel has become a voice for those who are afflicted by illness as well as for those who feel voiceless. I believe that readers will find understanding, wisdom, hope, and strength within her testimony.

Pastor Habte Adane
Dallas, America

Life is indeed a tapestry woven with various events and obstacles. However, a beautiful conclusion is attainable through sincere belief in God. It is my prayer that all believers finish their life race with grace and strength. The book addresses the author's journey through health challenges, showcasing how her steadfast faith and positive outlook have enabled her to navigate extraordinary circumstances successfully.

I have the privilege of knowing the author personally, as she is a voluntary supporter of our charity, EXCEL Family and Youth Society. Her pride in her culture, kind heart, and dedication to helping others are truly commendable. I admire her willingness to share her life story, as it speaks to the fact that our current situation does not dictate our future. This book addresses serious issues while demonstrating how individuals can overcome obstacles through unwavering faith and a renewed mindset.

Dr. Girma LuLu
Investment Officer & President, EXCEL Family and Youth Society
President

In the book titled "Love Letter," the author, Wongel , shares practical advice and insights drawn from her personal trials, demonstrating how she has lived according to the word of God. She addresses important themes such as overcoming challenges and provides principles that can guide readers in their own lives.

Many find her practical wisdom to be inspiring and applicable to their situations.

Readers are encouraged to approach this book with the understanding that it offers valuable insights, presented in simple English, much like those found in more scholarly works. It provides meaningful knowledge that can resonate just as powerfully as that from academic research or writings by highly educated authors.

Take the time to absorb the significant lessons within these pages, as the author shares not only her personal experiences but also extraordinary ideas that may challenge your perceptions. This book aims to illuminate truths that have long been present within her, and it offers an opportunity for growth and understanding.

Pastor Workneh Mogesse
Senior Pastor of Calgary Philadelphia Church

I was moved to tears while reading Wongel's book. It truly inspires the heart. I am confident that this book will positively impact many people's lives. I feel immensely blessed by your work and want to thank you for being a blessing to us.

Pastor Naod (Calgary, Canada)

Through the book "Love Letter," I have gained insights into the complexities of suffering faced by Christians. It has become clear that attributing their hardships solely to curses and sin can be unbiblical and disheartening for those experiencing difficulties. I recognize the importance of offering comfort and encouragement to individuals in need, rather than condemning them for their circumstances. I urge contemporary ministers to reflect on their teachings in this area and to anchor their messages in the truths found in God's Word. "Love Letter" has taught me the value of refraining from judgment toward those who are physically or mentally unwell. Instead, we should strive to support and uplift them, avoiding misinterpretation of Scripture that leads to condemnation.

(Auntie) Engudye Fantaw

After reading the remarkable book titled "Love Letter," I want to express my thoughts as one of your cousins who knows your story. Through this book, I've learned about your strength in many ways. Your determination not to give up in the face of life's struggles, combined with your ability to smile and persevere through trials, is truly inspiring. I am proud of you.
Sincerely,

Selam Fentaw (America)

We have found this book to be filled with educational, motivating, and encouraging advice. The author, Wongel Gebeyehu, challenges us by sharing her life experiences, which reflect her ups and downs alongside the word of God. We believe it serves as a wake-up call to get back on track, live a healthy Christian life, and persevere in our faith without faltering during times of tribulation. We can confidently say that a wide range of knowledge can be acquired by reading this book.
Sincerely,

Getachew (Dada) and Emebet (Chiye)
Nashville, Tennessee

The word of our God in Proverbs 12:26 says, "One who is righteous is a guide to his neighbor, but the way of the wicked leads them astray." I would like to thank the author for sharing her life experiences, allowing others to learn from them. I have known Wongel for over 15 years as a friend and for more than 8 years as my children's Sunday school teacher.

Her obedience and commitment to the Lord have comforted the hearts of many parents and members of the church. "Love Letter," apart from her childhood experiences, encapsulates the life she has practically lived in her hometown among us. Her life is filled with love, mercy, and a desire to benefit her community. I thank my Lord Jesus Christ for her and for the amazing gift of her book, which records her reliance on God during her treatment in a language that our children can understand. I believe that readers will greatly benefit from this book.

Rahel (Canada)

Wongel is my childhood friend, and I can attest that her family, as described in this book, embodies love and respect for people, treats everyone equally, and supports those in need. One notable aspect of Wongel's mother was her habit of greeting anyone from our neighborhood she encountered while driving; she would always get out of her car to say hello. I have observed this same kindness in Wongel.

This book addresses many serious issues and shares her insights from her experiences in a way that is easy to understand. It is particularly beneficial for cancer patients, individuals suffering from various forms of depression, and those whose families or friends are going through hardships. The book offers guidance on raising children, emphasizes walking in love within the house of God, and provides hope to those who may feel hopeless.

Selam Zelalem (Minnesota, USA)

Appreciation

Pastor workneh I would like to express my heartfelt gratitude to Pastor Workneh and his lovely wife, Masho. I have known them for a long time, and they have been a source of support during challenging times when I felt lost and unsure about my life. Their prayers and counsel have served as invaluable guidance, and they have been positive role models for me. Their constant support has helped me navigate the ups and downs of life, and they play a significant role in my journey. They have never judged me but have always encouraged me, becoming an integral part of my family. Thank you for being there for me through both the highs and lows, and for your uplifting words and love. I truly appreciate you both.

Pastor/singer Tekeste Getnet I would like to express my gratitude to Pastor Tekeste Getnet. Although we met only once during the conference, he was willing to assist me with my book. He took the initiative to connect me with important people and did everything he could to help. Pastor Tekeste genuinely wants to see others succeed and tirelessly supports those around him. I sincerely appreciate his ongoing assistance and the thoughtful answers he provides to my questions. Thank you very much, and may God bless you. Pastor Tekeste

Gene Beyene I would like to express my gratitude to Gene Beyene for her remarkable personality and the support she has provided me. She has consistently gone above and beyond, and her admiration for my beauty and style is a unique experience for me. Gene has been a source of encouragement in helping me navigate various challenges in life. When I celebrated my cancer-free day, she kindly invited everyone to join in the celebration. Her genuine desire to see others succeed has fostered mutual support between us through different obstacles. Thank you, Gene. I appreciate all that you have done.

kuku I would like to express my gratitude to my friend Ethiopia Rundassa, also known as Kuku, who is both my hiking companion and gym trainer. I appreciate her free spirit, which is truly contagious. Despite her busy schedule, she always makes time to meet with me when I ask. Kuku provides admiration and encouragement, and we have meaningful discussions on a variety of topics. We support each other during challenging times. As a trainer, she shares valuable tips on exercise and maintaining a balanced lifestyle. Her uplifting spirit and constant smile are genuinely appreciated.

Paulette, I want to take a moment to express my gratitude for your unwavering support as my best friend. You have consistently been there for me, offering prayers and encouragement when I needed them most. Whether during joyful moments or challenging times, your presence has been a source of strength.

During my cancer journey, your encouragement to write my book, despite facing your own challenges, was particularly meaningful. Thank you for being my inspiration and for everything you have done. I truly appreciate you.

Girmachew Habtie I would like to express my gratitude to Girmachew for his invaluable guidance and advice regarding my book. He has consistently offered his support without any judgment. Even during moments of frustration with certain aspects of my writing, he maintained a positive outlook and encouraged me to focus on possibilities rather than the negatives. He has also connected me with the right people, which has been incredibly helpful. I truly admire his encouraging attitude and his determination not to give up. I am immensely thankful for all the support he has provided, day and night. Your willingness to assist me every step of the way means a great deal to me. Thank you very much—I appreciate everything you have done for me.

Yonas Gezahegn I would like to acknowledge Yonas Gezahegn for his significant contribution to my work. Although I have not had the opportunity to contact him by phone or meet him in person, he was chosen for this project through Girmachew Habtie. Yonas played an important role in making the English-language version of the book available to readers by translating it from Amharic to English with a beautiful flow of language. His efforts are greatly appreciated.

Acknowledgement

First and foremost, I would like to express my gratitude to God for His guidance and care throughout my life. He has been with me during challenging times, especially when I faced serious health issues.

I am also thankful to my family for their sacrifices and support. They dedicated their time to comfort, encourage, and pray for me. When they had concerns, they communicated them with compassion. I appreciate their presence and support.

I want to express my deepest gratitude to my husband, Tsegish, who went above and beyond to support me during my battle with cancer. He was my rock, helping me through every moment when I couldn't even walk or lift a glass to drink water.

He supported me, prayed for me, and took care of the kids. He prepared them for school and took them to their activities while managing his own work. It was not easy, but he handled it all with grace and strength.

I would also like to thank my wonderful kids for their good behavior and for supporting me in everything I needed. May God bless you abundantly.

Friew I would like to express my gratitude to my spiritual mentor, Firew, who has passed on. He played a significant role in my spiritual growth since my early childhood, offering prayers and guidance. I also extend my appreciation to his wife, Yishamu, and their children who reside in America.

Abebaw The other person worthy of my appreciation is Abebaw. who played a pivotal role in my spiritual growth during my adolescence, a time when I faced significant challenges and caused concern for my family. I was struggling with anxiety, and my family didn't know how to help me. Abebaw stepped in, praying for me and offering loving support.

He helped my mother through prayer and guided me onto a positive path. He introduced me to Jesus in a profound way, preaching the word of God, teaching me the Bible, and showing me how to connect with the Almighty. He never gave up on me. Thank you, Abebaw, for helping me develop my relationship with Jesus and for being a true Christian who supports those struggling, especially teenagers like myself. Your efforts to rescue me during my tough times mean so much. May God bless you and your beautiful family abundantly.

Fantaw I am grateful to my former tutor, Fantaw who currently resides in Belgium. During the times I struggled to understand my school subjects, he provided valuable tutoring and support. His encouragement and motivation during moments when I felt hopeless made a significant difference. I will always remember his advice to believe in myself. Thank you, Fantaw

Ewnet Tedla I would like to extend my heartfelt thanks to Ewnet Tedla for playing a significant role in editing my book. I wrote this book by hand, using 35 pens to complete 279 pages, and her assistance was invaluable. She corrected all my handwriting, which was challenging to read, and typed out a copy of the manuscript. Additionally, she translated some sentences from English into Amharic. I am truly grateful for her patience and dedication in completing this task despite the difficulties presented by my handwriting. Thank you, Ewnet Tedla

Pastor Meron I would like to thank Pastor Meron for your incredible support during my difficult times. Your willingness to pray with me and accompany me to hospital appointments meant a lot. I also appreciate your beautiful wife, Tina, for being there for me as well. Together, you both provided encouragement and companionship when I needed it most.

Pastor Meron's dedication to sharing the gospel and spreading the love of Jesus in the community is truly inspiring, as he actively preaches not only from the pulpit but also on the streets. Additionally, I am grateful for the time he devoted to reviewing and providing constructive feedback on my book during its preparation. His support has been invaluable. Thank you once again for everything, and may God bless you and your family.

Evangelist Mekonen Demissie I would like to acknowledge Evangelist Mekonnen Demissie for his essential role in connecting me with the right people and ensuring a smooth editing process for my book. He was the first to believe in its potential and reassured me that many readers would appreciate it. His support during moments of doubt was invaluable, often

23

encouraging me with, "Wongel, you can do it; I will be there for you to the end." He was also proactive in addressing conflicts as they arose. I thank you, my brother Mekonnen, and your beautiful wife a million times for your significant contributions. May you be blessed abundantly.

Dr. Girma LuLu is a remarkable person who consistently provides positive motivation. He acknowledges even the smallest of my successes, which has greatly boosted my confidence. Recognizing my potential, he encourages me not to be limited by my environment.

Aware of my aspirations beyond possibly becoming a "fashion show" director, he has created opportunities for my growth. Though I faced setbacks with my dream in Paris, his encouragement has been unwavering. He was the first to offer me a platform to showcase my traditional garments to various countries, and I received my first certificate from him.

Dr. Girma has also motivated countless Ethiopian and Eritrean young adults to pursue their dreams and has provided support to those in need. His ongoing encouragement has inspired many to realize their potential and strive for their goals. I feel fortunate to have been a part of your organization and am grateful for all your support. Thank you, and may you be abundantly blessed.

Pastor Habte Adane, Thank you for your dedication and inspiration. Your deep love for God and your impactful preaching resonate with many around the world. I have learned valuable lessons from you, particularly the importance of keeping my focus on God and remaining steadfast through adversity. Your determination and commitment to the church are truly motivating.

I also appreciate your approachable personality and the lighthearted moments you bring after church programs. Your ability to make others laugh has made it easy to approach you. Thank you for being a source of motivation. Wishing you and your family abundant blessings.

Selam Zelalem I want to take a moment to acknowledge the significance of our friendship and express my heartfelt gratitude. You have played an important role in my life since childhood, and I cherish the memories we created together—our walks hand in hand, the letters we exchanged, and the messages delivered through friends in our neighborhood. Those times hold a special place in my heart.

Even as life led us in different directions, your visit during my battle with cancer truly touched me. Your support during that challenging time meant a great deal, and having you by my side at my appointments, praying and encouraging me, provided immense comfort.

Thank you for being a steadfast presence in my life. Your unwavering support has been invaluable to me. I thank you for being my rock and the person to whom I resort when I face problems and grow weary. The unshakeable support which you have rendered to me since your childhood has benefited me. I appreciate everything you have done, and I wish you and your family many blessings.

God bless you and your family. I thank you more than words can tell.

Richo Manaya I want to take a moment to express my heartfelt appreciation for your friendship and support over the years. Your presence in my life has been invaluable, especially during challenging times.

When I made mistakes, your non-judgmental advice guided me, and in moments when I felt low, you were always there. I will never forget how you supported me during my chemotherapy and the struggles I faced with swelling in my leg. Despite being pregnant with your third child, you took the time to massage my leg, showing your unwavering determination to help me feel better.

Your daily visits to the hospital, along with the prayers shared by you and your family, were incredibly comforting. You went out of your way to invite me to your home and even took me to a restaurant, which brought me joy during a difficult period. Your constant encouragement and reminders that I would see light in the darkness were truly uplifting.

Thank you for everything you have done for me. I wish you and your family abundant blessings.

Achalu Bire (Real Estate Agent) I would like to extend my sincere thanks to Achalu Bire (Real Estate Agent)and his wife Emuti. Throughout my journey to complete this book, their encouragement and financial support were invaluable. I am truly grateful for their ongoing assistance with the various needs that arose during this process. May God bless you both abundantly.

Chuni has been an incredibly supportive friend during my illness. Her presence was a constant source of strength; she visited me in the hospital and cooked meals for me when I needed them. No matter what I required, she was always there to help. Through both my highs and lows, she provided encouragement, prayers, and valuable advice. Chuni also motivated me to pursue writing a book and offered financial support for this endeavor. Her significant contributions to this project have been invaluable, and I am truly grateful for everything she has done. Thank you, Chuni. Wishing you abundant blessings.

Mekonnen Adamu I would like to extend special thanks to the editor of this book, Mekonnen Adamu. I am amazed at your patience, prayer and encouragement in the course of this work.
I thank you for believing in me and taking the responsibility of the editorial work. Particularly, since my first manuscript was written in extremely simple Amharic, it was not easy to translate the English version, which was also written by me, into good Amharic. Even then you have done everything to support me. I am sincerely grateful for your doing whatever you could to

support me; you did not give up on me. God bless you and your wonderful family.

I thank all the people who visited me while I was struggling with my cancer. Some of them brought food to my house,

while some others came to my house and prayed for me. There were some friends who, apart from encouraging me, wept with me while accompanying me to my appointment. I have tremendous admiration for all believers who brought me flowers and took me to restaurants. Most of you have visited me at the hospital. I thank all those who were there for me in my ups and downs. I will never forget your kindness and compassion. It is my wish you received innumerable blessings.

I would also like to thank Pastor Anthony Greco who supported me a lot and Paulette Winsor who helped me a lot with everything I needed. I thank you, Aileen Werner, Maddi, Selina, for your goodness.

I would like to thank brother Apostle Petros sincerely for working on the interior page layout and cover design diligently.

Finally, my heartfelt thanks goes to Pastor Meron Woldehawariat, Pastor Habte Adane, Pastor Workneh Mogese, Evangelist Mekonen Demissie, Pastor Tewodros Chernet, Pastor Naod, Doctor Girma Bekele, Richo Manaya

Enguday Fentaw, Selam Fentaw, Getachew and Embet who have read my book and given me constructive comments. God Most High bless you all.

Why Is It Important to Write This Book?

It is an undeniable fact that each of us will eventually depart from this world, prompting an important question: What legacy will we leave for future generations? I firmly believe in the value of documenting the experiences I have navigated—the triumphs and setbacks, along with the lessons learned—so that others may derive wisdom from them. This conviction inspired me to write this book, with the hope that readers will uncover meaningful insights within its pages.

Oprah Winfrey once remarked, "Nothing that you have been through will be wasted." This serves as a poignant reminder that even when we struggle to comprehend the significance of our challenges, they can offer valuable lessons to others.

I have personal motivations for writing this book. Firstly, I aim to encourage my readers and help them regain hope in difficult situations. I also wish to provide solace to those affected by cancer, reassuring them that they are not alone in their suffering. My journey through this illness has shown me that, like myself, they too can emerge from their trials and ultimately find the strength to support others.

Additionally, I want to highlight the protection, mercy, and kindness that I have experienced from God throughout my journey. I believe this book will offer comfort to those facing various challenges and instill a sense of hope in their hearts.

Writing this book has been a lengthy journey for me, spanning many years. Throughout this process, I have experienced significant loss, as several close friends and family members have passed away. These were individuals who provided comfort and support during my struggles, including my biological father and spiritual father, as well as friends who reached out through social media. Their absence left a void in my life, and at times, I found myself overwhelmed by grief, feeling discouraged and contemplating whether to continue writing.

Compounding these feelings were the challenges of time constraints and various obstacles that made the path to publication seem daunting. Yet, amid these trials, I felt the unwavering guidance of the Holy Spirit encouraging me to persevere. I believe that sharing my story can help others witness God's healing power and offer them comfort in their own struggles. This conviction has motivated me to complete this book, emphasizing its importance as a source of hope and encouragement for those in similar situations.

I have chosen the title "Love Letter" for my book to express my intention of sharing my life experiences with my readers in a spirit of compassion and connection. I sincerely hope that you find both enjoyment and insight in your reading.

Enjoy your reading!
Wongel Gebeyehu
May 2025.

31

Introduction

I would like to share my story to encourage those who have recently been diagnosed with cancer and those currently undergoing treatment. I firmly believe that my experiences can provide comfort and inspire others to cope with this illness. Throughout my journey, I have encountered many individuals facing various types of cancer. When I share my story, many express that it motivates them, and some have told me that it has given them hope and strength. My deepest desire is to inspire others to fight against cancer.

During my time as a cancer patient, I struggled with feelings of shame and isolation. I often felt embarrassed about my appearance, which led me to avoid social interactions. The cancer greatly weakened me, making it impossible for me to walk, dress, or care for myself without assistance. The effects of chemotherapy were harsh; my skin suffered, my nails turned black, and I experienced persistent swelling in my tongue and throat. The weekly injections I received took a toll on my body. Throughout my battle with cancer, I underwent 11 major surgeries. On one occasion, a 16-hour surgery led to complications, and it seemed as though I might not survive the procedure.

During those challenging times, I often isolated myself from everyone, including my family. It was incredibly difficult not wanting anyone to see me in that state. Yet, despite these struggles, I emerged stronger. I am a warrior. I am a survivor. I am a woman who has faced these hardships and triumphed.

My journey as a cancer patient was filled with challenges, but my Lord Jesus Christ remained by my side throughout. He never left me. He granted me rest, peace, faith, and hope. Through His strength and grace, I found the resilience to face each day. While I encountered many trials and turbulent moments, I can confidently affirm that my Lord, who loves me, has never abandoned me in difficult times. I hope my story encourages you to confront any challenges you may face. Remember, with God, nothing is impossible.

This book is organized into 31 chapters, each of which can be read independently.

Chapter One

A Glimpse into the Past

1. The Sad Stories

I wish to begin my narrative by taking a journey back to my childhood. I was fortunate to be born into a loving and well-educated family that valued respect and support for others. My mother, a graduate of Addis Ababa University, dedicated over three decades to the Economic Commission for Africa (ECA). Her career required her to travel extensively, allowing her to immerse herself in diverse cultures. Renowned for her elegance, she always dressed impeccably.

Similarly, my father served our nation as a diplomat during the 1980s, stationed in the former Soviet Union. He represented Ethiopian students living in Eastern Europe and, in the 1990s, took on the role of Deputy Delegate of Ethiopia to UNESCO in Paris. Following his tenure there, he returned to Ethiopia, where he worked as an education advisor. He played a vital role in advocating for the care of children from an early age and in shaping educational policy.

Throughout my upbringing, my parents devoted themselves to my well-being, ensuring that I received the nurturing and guidance I needed.

Although I grew up without wanting for anything and had all my needs met, I could not dismiss the troubling questions that lingered in my mind. I vividly recall days when I was consumed by the thought, "Why are other children suffering from hunger, lacking basic necessities, while I live comfortably without any deprivation?"

As I transitioned from childhood into adolescence, these questions became even more pronounced. Witnessing the suffering of others, hearing their stories, and seeing children begging on the streets filled me with sadness and heartbreak. At times, I would weep uncontrollably. I often questioned, "Why do such hardships happen to women and children?"

In our neighborhood, there were both wealthy and poor families. My mother was a deeply spiritual woman who dedicated her time to praying with anyone, regardless of their economic status, and was committed to helping those in need. Her spiritual dedication was well-known among the believers in our community. Upon returning home from work, her first priority—before even changing her clothes—was to spend time in prayer with those who sought her support. After listening to their prayer requests, she prayed for them earnestly and often provided financial assistance. Feeding the hungry and clothing the needy were core principles that guided her daily life.

People who came to share their stories with my mother often had to wait for her to return from the office. During that time, I approached some of them to inquire about their struggles. Many told me, "You're still a kid; you can't understand our concerns." However, a few did share their thoughts with me. After hearing their stories, I would close my bedroom door and pray earnestly for them.

I prayed earnestly to God, saying, "Jesus Christ, please put an end to the hardships faced by these people. Why do these difficulties befall those who believe in You? Why don't you visit them soon?" My mother was aware of the questions I posed to the Lord during my prayers. She reminded me that God does not ask "Why?"; He knows the reasons behind His actions. However, I viewed God as a close relative and felt compelled to ask Him "Why?" Despite my persistent inquiries, I received no answer.

One of my neighbors had a large compound, but her house was still incomplete. She had a seven-year-old child and twins, and her husband was the sole provider for the family.

She was uneducated and did not have a job, relying entirely on her husband's income to care for her household. I became acquainted with her when she came to my mother for prayer. One day, her husband suddenly vanished, leaving her to care for their children alone. She was overwhelmed and confused, unsure of how to navigate the drastic changes that had occurred in her life. When she came to share her situation with my mother, my mother had not yet returned from work.

She sat in our living room, awaiting my mother, tears streaming down her face as her children cried alongside her. I felt compelled to understand the reason for her distress, so I approached her and asked, "What happened?"

She explained, "It has been two weeks since my husband abandoned us, and we have not had anything to eat during that time. My children are hungry. Today, two unknown men came to our house and said, 'Leave our house. Your husband has sold the land to us. Here's proof.' They showed me a piece of paper. I fell to their feet, pleading with them not to evict us for the sake of my children. I asked, 'Where will we go?' They responded that I had one month to find a new place to live. That is why I came here for prayer."

Hearing her story filled me with sorrow.

I will never forget the tears streaming down her face. I found myself asking, "Why do such hardships befall people?" Without hesitation, I ensured that she and her children were served food. While she waited for my mother, I retreated to my bedroom to pray, my heart heavy with concern.

One day, a woman named Tsehay came to our house seeking prayer because she had a wound on her forehead. I asked, surprised, "What happened to you?"

She explained, "Someone knocked on our gate, and when I opened it, an unknown man struck me on the forehead with a stone."

I inquired, "What did you do to provoke him? Do you know who he is?"

She shook her head, saying, "I don't know him. He ran away after injuring me."

I suggested, "Take our guard with you. You need to find a way to address this situation. Who would care for your children if something worse happened to you? Having our guard with you might intimidate him."

She replied, "You're being unrealistic. I came here to pray with your mother."

I felt a surge of anger at the injustice of the situation, muttering to myself, "What right does someone have to harm another without reason? People can be robbed or even killed." My father noticed my agitation and asked, "Are you praying?"

Without answering his question, I bombarded him with my inquiries. "Why do people treat others unfairly? Why do they inflict pain on others? Such individuals should be held accountable. Why is it that the rights of victims are not protected? When will their rights be safeguarded?"
He responded, "For now, I don't have answers to your questions, but have you considered discussing these issues with your brothers? Worrying about someone else's plight doesn't help either of us resolve the current problems."

I replied, "I want to become a crime investigator. I will make it my mission to apprehend every criminal and ensure they are punished. I will prove this to you when I grow up." My father smiled and said, "That's a very good idea."

2. The Little Girl Whose Life Was Cut Short

When I was a student, I knew a girl whom I cared for deeply. She often came to school with bruises on her face. I would ask her, "What happened to your face?" and she would reply, "My mother beat me for getting 80 marks on my exam. My father comes home drunk and beats my mother and me." When I inquired why they hurt her, she said, "I would be happy if I knew the reason."

This little girl was only ten years old when she passed away. The school was informed that "she committed suicide." This raised a question for me: "How can a ten-year-old girl commit suicide?" There was a chapel on the school grounds where we would go to pray whenever we faced issues or difficulties. After praying, we would leave the chapel and return to our usual activities, just like other children.

During our time together, this girl had never expressed any intention of taking her own life. I knew her well, and despite the verbal and physical abuse she endured, she had never mentioned thoughts of suicide. Instead, I remember her saying, "I will go to my aunt or my grandfather" when she could no longer tolerate her home situation. I suspect that her death may have occurred during an incident of violence she experienced.

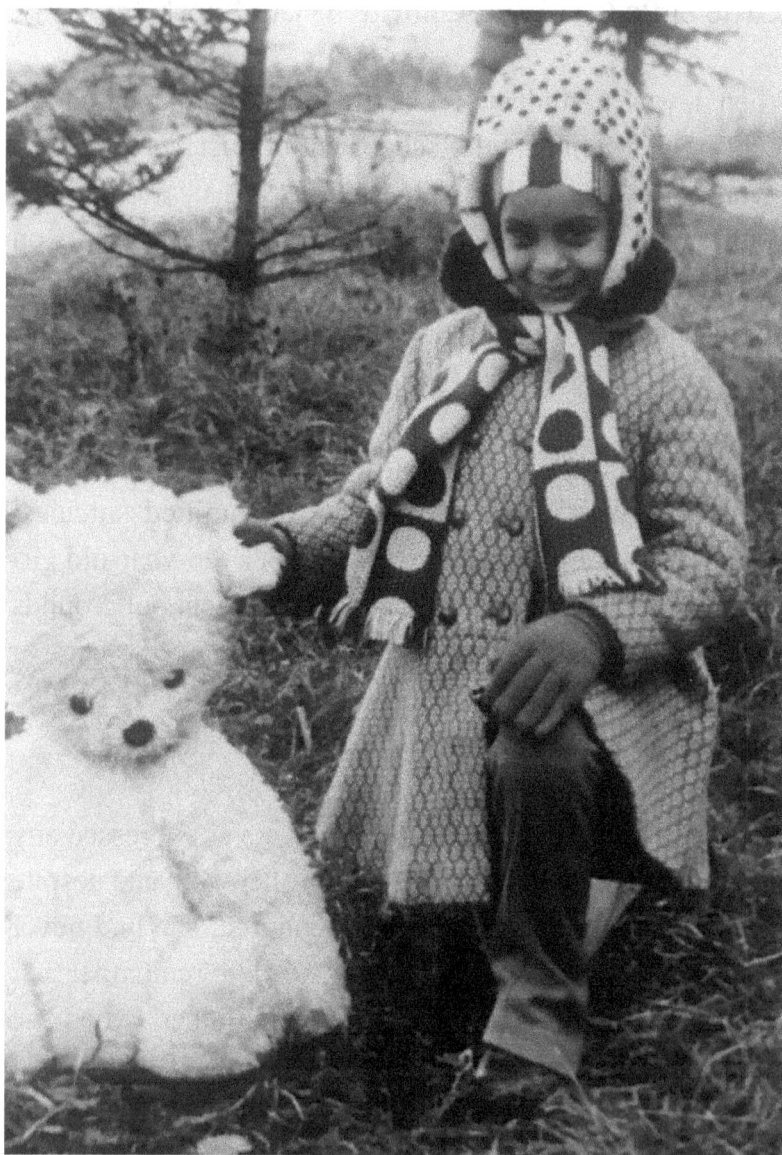

I sometimes shared my suspicions with another girl I knew. The sadness from the girl's passing weighed heavily on my mind, prompting me to say, "I want to have this matter investigated." I asked this girl to accompany me to the deceased's home, expressing my desire to speak with her parents. She smiled and responded, "Who do you think you are to interview her mother and father?"

I replied, "I am a crime investigator." She cautioned me against proceeding, saying, "You're not a crime investigator yet. If you go and invite them for an interview, they might not take you seriously because you're a child; they could even react aggressively." She added, "Why get involved in someone else's issues at such a young age?" Her remarks discouraged me from pursuing the visit.

3. My Desire to Become a Crime Investigator

That night, while I was kneeling in prayer, I expressed a desire to my Lord: "In the future, I want to work on human rights for women and children in this country. Alternatively, since my parents are well-educated, I could encourage them to establish such an organization." After finishing my prayer, I reflected on my long-standing dream of becoming a homicide detective. I resolved, "I want to become a prosecutor."

I remember being in France when the O.J. Simpson case gained widespread attention. I was captivated by the story and watched coverage day and night, much to the frustration of my father and brothers, who eventually hid the remote control. I was eagerly anticipating the verdict, and before he was declared innocent, I believed he was guilty. I told my brother, "O.J. Simpson is guilty," to which he responded, "You're being racist; you should support him simply because he is black." I clarified that my stance was not about race, but rather about truth. I believed he was 95 percent guilty, although he had prominent lawyers representing him. I have maintained my opinion on this matter; I still believe he was guilty and felt disappointed by the outcome of the trial.

I referenced the O.J. Simpson case to illustrate my strong desire to become a prosecutor. This deep interest in criminal justice has led me to regularly watch various television programs that explore these themes. Notable shows I enjoy include Dateline, Unsolved Mysteries, True Crime, and 20/20. I find these channels compelling because they focus on issues of justice. Some of the specific cases that have captured my attention include Jodi Arias, Making a Murderer, Steven Avery, the Mendez Brothers, and JonBenét Ramsey. I have great admiration for Nancy Grace, as I appreciate her ability to bring attention to criminal cases and advocate for justice.

From her work, I have learned a great deal, which has further fueled my desire to advocate for victims.

I also want to mention that I admire several "YouTubers" who share true crime stories. Among them are Eleanor Neale, Kendall Rae, Danelle Hallan, and Christina Randall. I find Christina particularly impactful due to her experiences and the insights she shares from her time in prison, which resonate with many viewers. Danelle Hallan's perspective is also valuable, and I appreciate Leya Nicole for her focus on praying for victims. Additionally, I follow Stephanie Harlowe, Jackie Flores from "60 Minutes in Australia," and "True Crime Every Day."

The YouTubers I follow include Stephanie Harlowe, Jackie Flores from "60 Minutes in Australia," and "True Crime Every Day," among others. It appears that the mentions of these YouTubers, TV shows, and Netflix documentaries were omitted due to concerns that readers might not have the time or interest to engage with them. However, I believe that many young readers of my English book will find these references valuable. Thank you for considering this!

YouTubers:

• Candace Owens
• Stephanie Soo

- Fumi Desalu-Vold

Documentaries:

- "Orlando Bloom: Meet Children Working in Bangladesh"
- "Daughter of Destiny"
- "Take Care of Maya"
- "Grizzly Man"
- "Grey Gardens"
- "The Last Day"
- "Mystery of Maya"
- "Sans Soleil" by Chris Marker
- "Grand Canyon: The Hidden Secrets"
- "La Marche de l'Empereur"
- "Unsolved Mysteries"
- "Who Killed JonBenét Ramsey?"
- "Red Zones: The World's Toughest Places"
- "The Discreet Lives of the Super Rich"

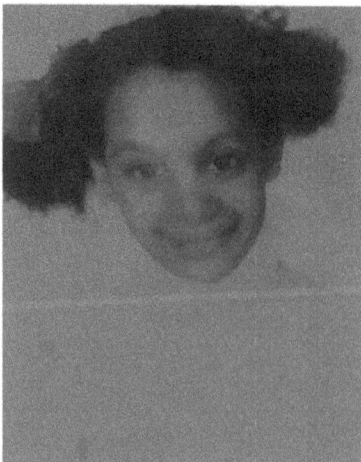

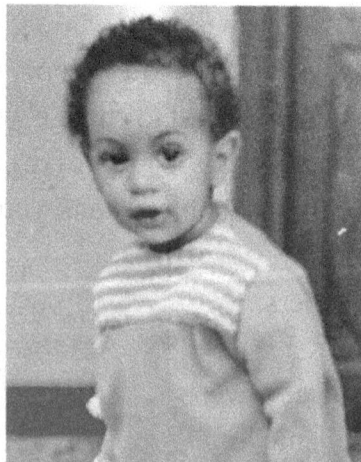

From a young age, I was eager to transition into adulthood and pursue a career as a crime investigator. My fascination with crime was sparked early on by stories of unforgettable crimes against individuals, often involving victims who had no support. I frequently pondered how I would navigate the challenges of investigating these crimes. My passion for this field only grew stronger over time. If asked, "What do you want to be in the future?" I would confidently respond, "A crime investigator."

However, when I shared this aspiration with a particular sister, her reaction was dismissive. She remarked, "This is primarily a man's job; it's not suitable for a woman." Unfortunately, I found little support for my dream from those around me.

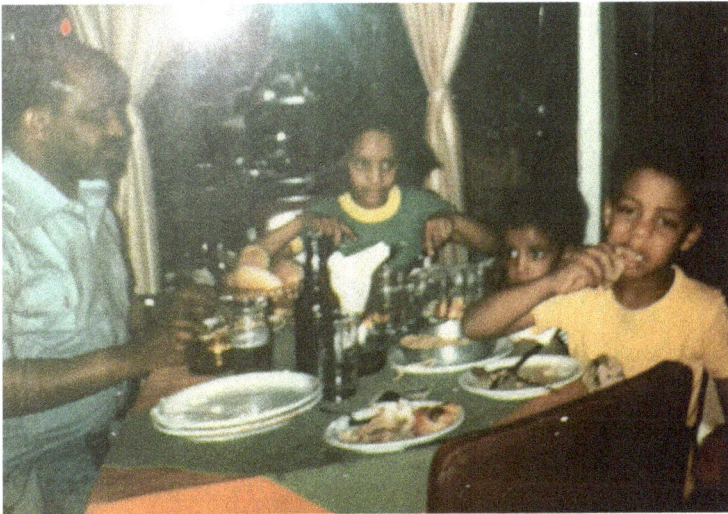

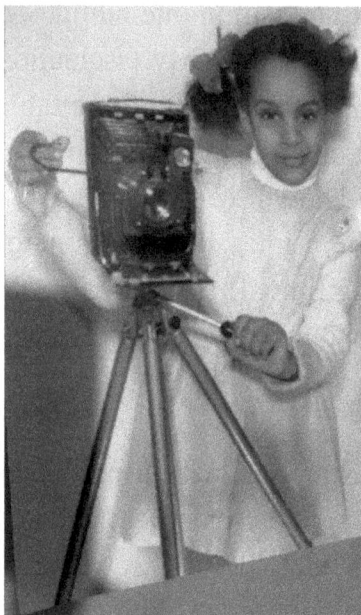
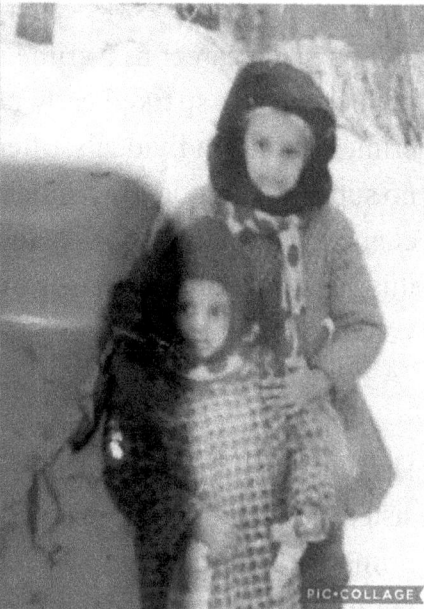

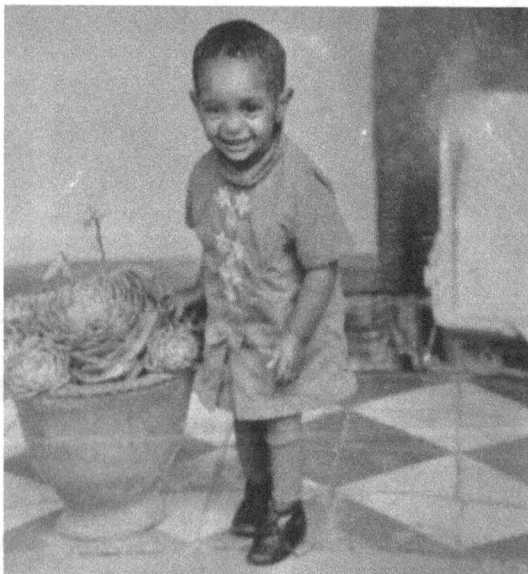

Chapter TWo

The Amazing Visitation of the Holy Spirit

1. The Hand of God Which Rescued the Young Child

During my childhood, I was a devoted girl of prayer, and I experienced the Lord's power in profound ways. When people entered my bedroom, they often felt overwhelmed by the presence of the Holy Spirit. While my parents were at work, I would gather the neighborhood children to pray with them and to share teachings. I also welcomed mothers into my room, where we would pray together when they visited to see my mother. Witnessing the Holy Spirit work through me filled me with awe, and I often prayed earnestly, saying, "Oh, Lord, if you can work through me, a young girl, in such a powerful manner, I aspire to be your instrument more as I grow older."

One day, I was watching a preacher named Pastor Benny Hinn on television, and I found myself saying, "Oh Lord, use me just like this man." This sparked an even greater thirst for the Spirit of the Lord in me, especially after reading his book, Good Morning, Holy Spirit.

Not long after, a mother came to our house with her child, who she claimed was dead. She requested that I pray for him despite my initial hesitation, as my mother was not home. The mother insisted, and I agreed. As soon as I laid my hand on the child, to my astonishment, he opened his eyes and began to cry and move. This miracle occurred following a prayer that lasted less than five minutes.

The mother knelt before me, expressing her gratitude by calling me an angel. I quickly redirected the praise, telling her, "It is Jesus who healed your son; it is in His name that I prayed. He alone deserves the honor and praise, so go home and thank the Lord."

The mother expressed her astonishment, saying, "The Lord is performing miracles through you. I came here because I heard people say that there is a praying girl here, and miracles always happen when she prays." I was taken aback, as I never expected God to use me, a young child, in such a significant way. I thought to myself, "I am going to become like Benny Hinn." As I witnessed the mercy, kindness, love, and faithfulness of the Lord, my connection to Him deepened, and my love and respect for Him grew.

The Lord gradually revealed to me that He has a purpose for everything, and He taught me more with each passing day.

One day, during class, my teacher posed a question: "What do you want to become?" When it was my turn, I confidently replied, "A crime investigator." Her reaction surprised me; she laughed heartily and said, "You are a child with learning difficulties. Just being promoted from one grade to the next is a miracle."

At that moment, I felt embarrassed and wished I could disappear. I struggled to hold back my tears as I noticed some of my classmates laughing. The teacher further commented, "I don't like students who aren't willing to acknowledge their limitations." Her words stung, causing my childhood dream of becoming a crime investigator to gradually fade away due to the discouragement I received from various places.

2. Inarticulacy (Alexithymia)

In regard to my learning pace, I wasn't a fast learner. When I was informed during my doctoral education that I had ADHD, I shared this with my father, who dismissed it, telling me not to discuss it further. As a result, I kept the issue to myself for a long time. The people around me often made fun of my stutter, making me anxious during conversations. I found it particularly challenging to engage with new people, which left me looking upset and confused.

However, amidst these struggles, I felt a reassuring presence from the Lord, who reminded me, "Just as I loosened Moses' tongue, so will I loosen your tongue. I will use you in a unique way." Alongside my stutter, I frequently found it difficult to express my ideas, which contributed to feelings of insecurity. Despite this, I experienced a sense of loving support from Jesus in dealing with all my challenges. I often found that my hands expressed more than my words could. When I wanted to communicate, I would gesture with both my hands and my mouth, relying heavily on my hands due to my speech impediment. Writing became my primary means of expression, leading me to produce a significant number of prayers, poems, and other works. Despite my stuttering, I believed that the Lord would use me and remove my speech challenges.

I experienced a deep sense of joy in my relationship with the Lord, feeling His presence and love surrounding me. I held onto the conviction that He would help me overcome my difficulties and bring glory to His name. Throughout my childhood, I often wondered how this transformation might occur, given my circumstances.

To my surprise, many people have shown me kindness, recognizing the favor of God in my life. I have built connections with others and enjoy praying with them, but I find even greater fulfillment in spending time alone with the Lord. I often dedicated entire days in my bedroom to prayer, finding solace in His presence.

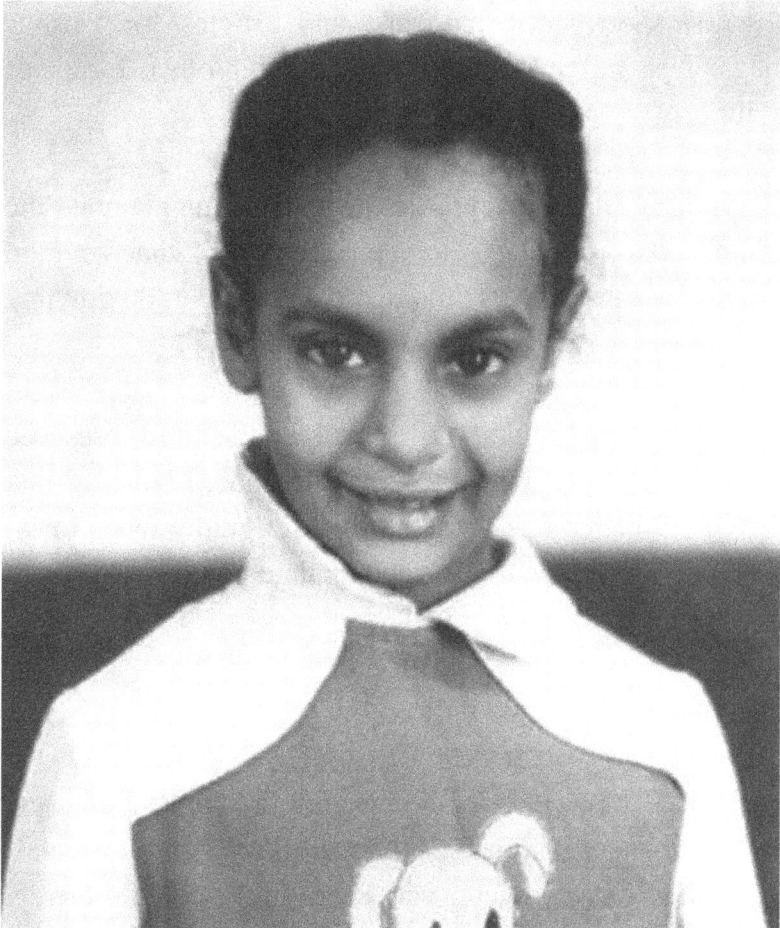

Communication for me often relied more on gestures than spoken words, as my speech impediment made verbal expression challenging. I would use a combination of hand movements and my voice to convey my thoughts, but writing became my primary outlet. I have written many prayers, short stories, poems, and articles for various magazines and newspapers, along with other forms of writing.

Despite my Inarticulacy (Alexithymia) i maintainned the belief that I could be used positively and that I would eventually find ways to overcome my (Alexithymia)difficulties.

This conviction brought me joy, as I felt the divine presence of the Lord in my life. Since my childhood, I believed that He would never forget me and would guide my journey, even as I questioned how such change could occur given my circumstances.

Interestingly, I found that many people were drawn to me, likely because of the positive influence of God's favor in my life. I have developed meaningful connections and enjoy praying with others, although I often find the greatest peace in solitary moments with the Lord. I would frequently spend entire days in my bedroom, engaged in prayer and reflection.

Chapter Three

I Discovered My Talent

1. Teaching Children

A strong desire has developed within me, gradually growing stronger over time. This desire is to become a teacher. After much anguish and despair, my ambition to become a crime investigator declined. However, I didn't want to abandon it altogether. So, I went to my doctor for consultation. As soon as I met him, I said, "What should I do? I must become a crime investigator, but I lack the motivation to join a university and study there."

My doctor replied, "You don't necessarily have to focus on just one path. For instance, I know you love teaching and are good at it." He then asked, "What do you find yourself doing most of the time?" I responded, "I often find myself gathering and teaching children. You know that I am currently teaching them."

He continued, "What else do you enjoy doing?" I answered, "I like baking cakes, designing clothes, engaging in artistic work, reading, and writing a book. But I always find myself teaching children and contemplating how I can expand my knowledge by joining a university and earning a degree."

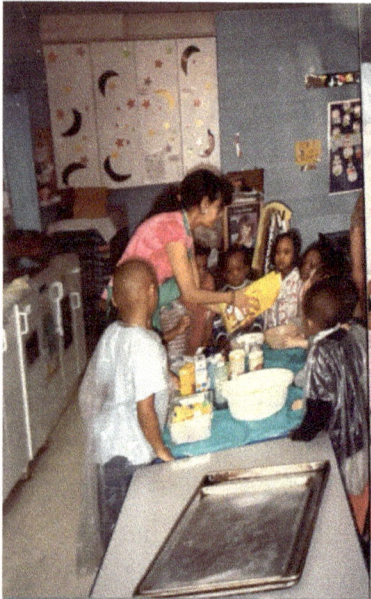

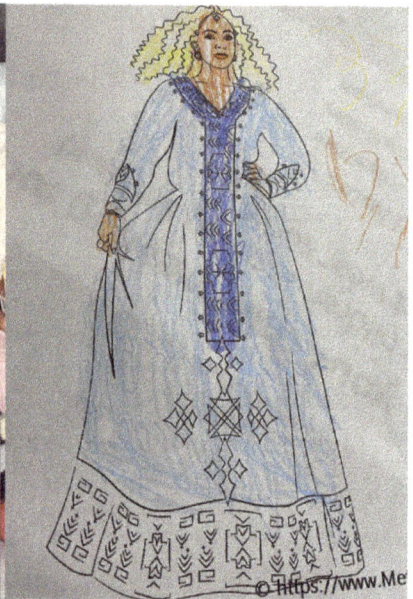

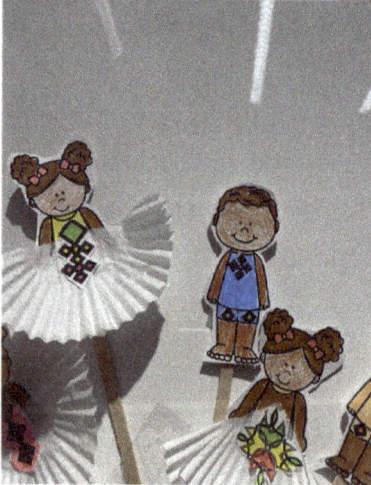

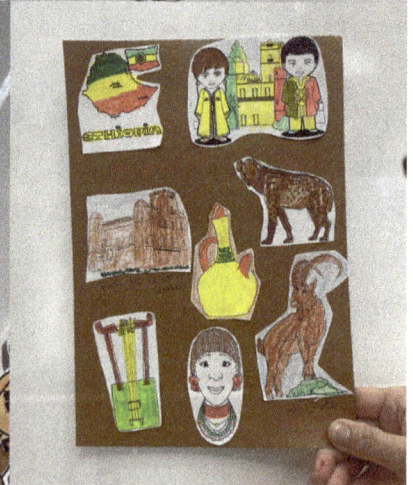

presents a picture that highlights efforts to introduce culture and heritage to students through Ethiopian crafts. It also notes the achievement of being the first woman to develop these crafts for children.

He said to me, "You can become a teacher, a child caregiver, a journalist, a copy editor, a beauty professional, or a hairdresser. People who experience similar challenges are often compassion-nate and generous; they tend to live for others. They have a strong desire to recover quickly and possess independent thinking. They are balanced and decisive, with qualities such as humor, love, innovation, trustworthiness, oratory skills, compassion, and steadfast-ness. They often have inspiring personalities. You don't have to become a crime investigator. Instead, you should consider taking courses to become a teacher. Once you achieve that, you can later pursue a career as a crime investigator."

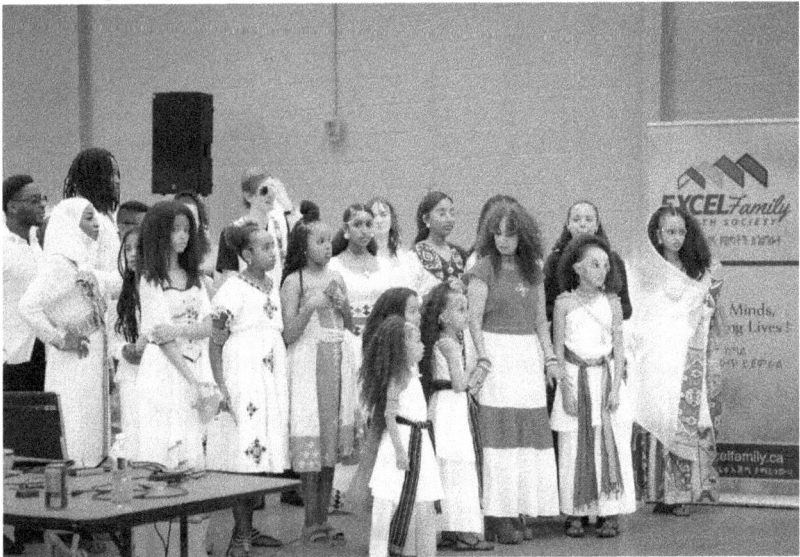

fundraising for kids at the fashion show.

While I was in France, I tried various pursuits, including courses in becoming a flight attendant, hospitality and tourism management, travel and tourism, and fashion design. However, my heart was set on becoming a lawyer. I took my doctor's advice seriously and started enrolling in courses to become a teacher.

I obtained my Early Childhood Education diploma and became a daycare teacher. Additionally, I have completed various courses, including child ADHD, child psychology, managing anger in children, classroom mental health, addressing sexual abuse to protect children, and childhood anxiety.

I started my career as a preschool teacher in a daycare, followed by a position as an assistant teacher in kindergarten. I also worked with children of all age groups at summer camps and after-school programs.

My experience includes working with children in various play areas and teaching Sunday school at my church. Overall, my life has revolved around working with children. After earning my diploma, I began teaching and working with kids, including those with special needs. This experience has provided me with valuable insights into their diverse backgrounds. I have had the opportunity to work with children from many countries,

including China,Philipian, Russia, Ukraine, Yugoslavia, Estonia,Finland,Greece India, Nigeria,Cameron kenya, zambia,   Eritrea, Morocco, Algeria, Germany, France, Bulgaria, Afghanistan, Korea, Japan, Italy, Romania, Slovakia Spain, Sweden Australia Vietnam, British, Brazil, Colombia, Mexico, Egypt, Hungary, Bangladesh, Haiti, Israel, Kazakhstan, and Pakistan, among others. I am grateful for each child I have encountered, as I have learned a great deal from them.

My life took an unexpected turn when I became a mother before completing my studies. Naturally, I devoted much of my time to caring for my children. I tend to focus intensely on tasks, which means I often struggle with multitasking.

This focus on motherhood left me little time for myself, leading to feelings of depression. Additionally, not being able to complete my studies created considerable psychological pressure. While I recognize that life has its ups and downs, I also believe that everything happens according to a greater plan. Despite the challenges I faced, I have seen moments of deliverance and support during difficult times.

As I mentioned earlier, my initial aspiration to become a crime investigator diminished. However, my desire to become a teacher grew stronger, prompting me to enroll in college and take courses to enhance my skills. Spending most of my time with children contributed to my difficulty in understanding adult conversations. I often found myself saying things directly, as I didn't hold onto grudges. My experiences with children taught me values such as meekness, kindness, and goodness. Teaching, playing, and

spending time with children brought me a unique sense of joy, and my love for them significantly increased. I spent around eight hours each day in their company.

Over time, I developed a child-like perspective that made adult communication challenging. For a long period, my closest friends were children. I also experienced periods of loneliness, during which I felt overlooked by others.

In these moments, I found a supportive presence in my faith. My relationship with my Lord Jesus Christ developed into a source of comfort. He understood my feelings and did not judge me, which drew me closer to Him. His joy and peace filled my life, and I felt an increased sense of favor.

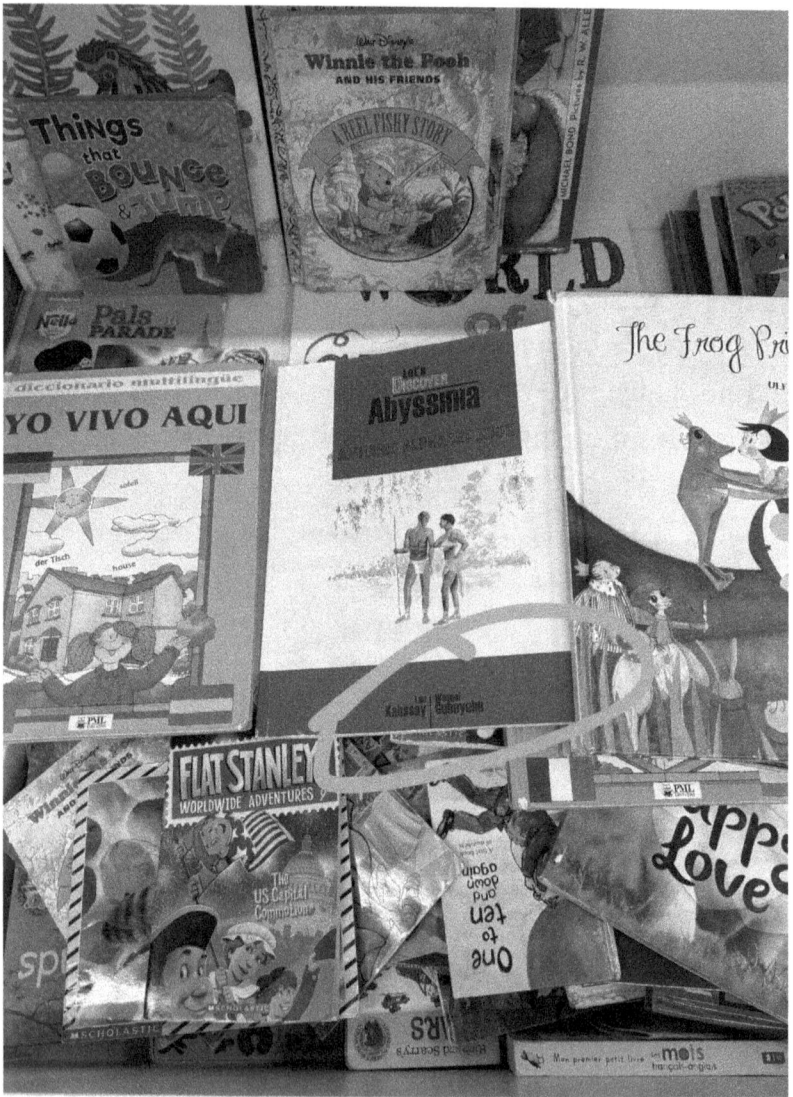

I have written a children's book that has sold out.

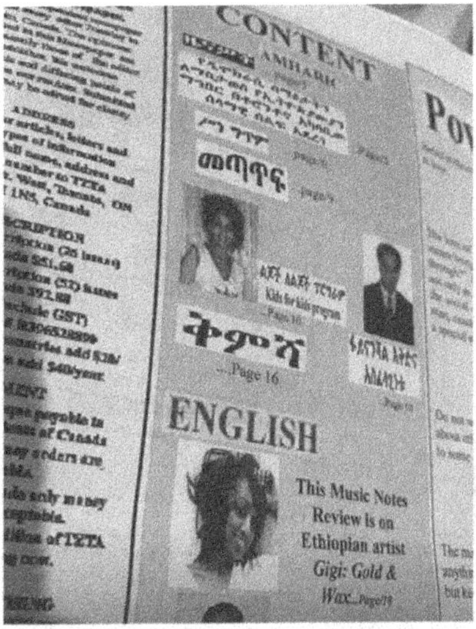

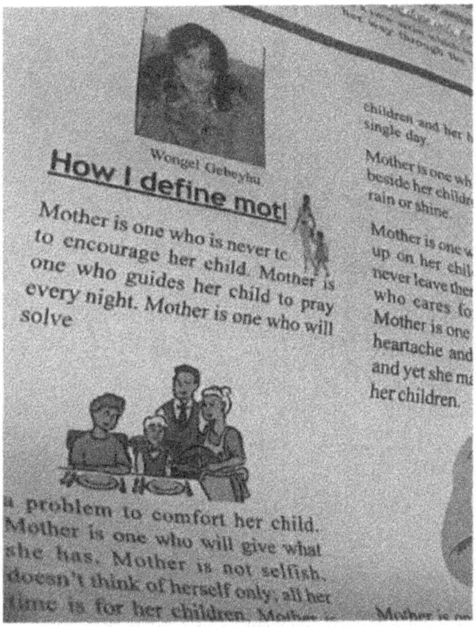

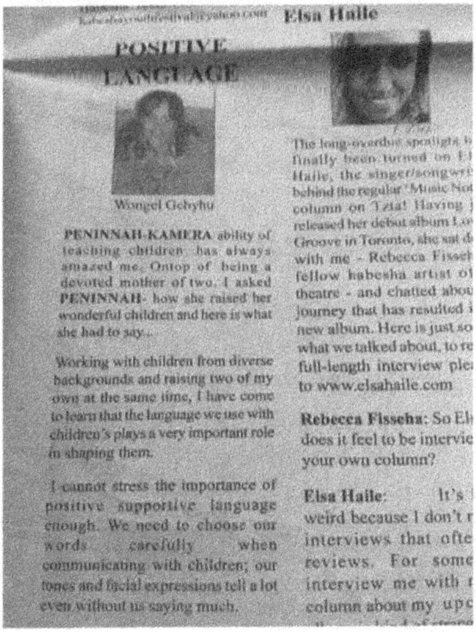

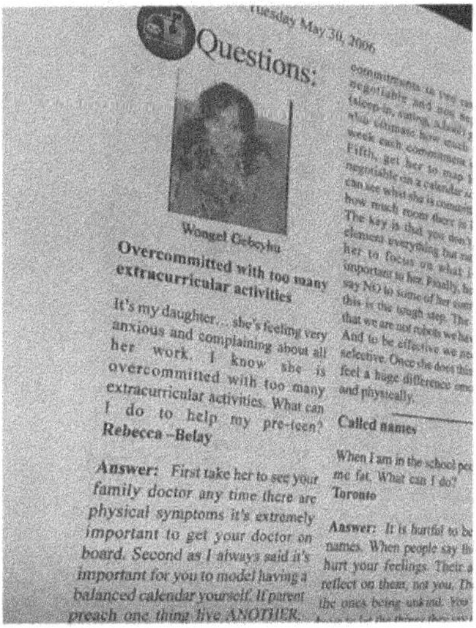

I used to write articles on various topics for a newspaper.

I used to write articles on various topics for a newspaper.

Chapter Four

I Became a Victim of Fear

1. My Peace Was Shaken

As I went through this difficult situation, I felt my heart racing unexpectedly, and I found myself crying for no apparent reason. The fear washed over me, and I sensed that I was engaged in a serious spiritual battle. I continued to pray earnestly, questioning, "Am I at risk of a car accident?" Anxiety and concern gripped me. I worried about the safety of my parents and family members. To ease my mind, I made frequent phone calls to confirm that they were all alright. Whenever the spirit of fear enveloped me, I resisted it vigorously, and, in those moments, a sense of peace would return. Unfortunately, this peace was often fleeting, and the fear would creep back in. I struggled to understand these feelings and found myself feeling quite confused.

2. The Symptoms Manifested

It had never occurred to me—nor had I even dreamt—that I would face health issues, so I rarely prayed about my health. I am quite cautious about what I eat and take various measures to maintain my well-being, including regular physical exercise.

Throughout my life, I have also been attentive to my family's dietary habits. Although I once experienced pneumonia, I had fully recovered long ago. My greatest fear has always been the prospect of being dependent on others due to illness, and I pray earnestly before God to protect me from such a situation. I do not wish to be a burden to anyone.

Despite my diligence in prayer, my fear persisted. Nevertheless, I held onto hope, continuing to pray that my children and I would remain under God's protection. One day, as I was leaving the swimming pool, a friend noticed something unusual on my body. With a surprised and concerned expression, she asked, "Have you seen a doctor?" I replied calmly, "No, I haven't." Later, I confirmed that there was indeed a change in my body, as she had pointed out. I undergo a thorough health checkup annually, and my doctor has reassured me that I have no health issues. I found myself questioning, "What is going on in my life?"

A friend encouraged me to see a doctor, so I made an appointment. After my examination, my doctor assured me that he had found no tumors in my body. Confused, I asked, "What then is the source of this concern?" He explained that sometimes such anomalies can occur and suggested that if it worsened, I could explore other treatment options.

On another occasion, while swimming with a few friends, two of them pointed out simultaneously, "Wongel, have you noticed the difference between your two breasts? They don't look the same." Their comments shocked me, prompting me to visit my doctor again. This time, I underwent an ultrasound, but again, nothing abnormal was found.

I underwent further examinations, but still, no issues were identified.

Despite being relieved by the absence of a diagnosis, I continued to feel inwardly troubled. One day, while preparing for a New Year dinner party, I asked my daughter to help me choose an outfit. While assisting me, she suddenly observed my breast and remarked, "There seems to be something wrong with your breast." I was taken aback, unsure of how to respond, and felt a wave of disturbance wash over me.

I attended my doctor's appointment and asked him to examine me thoroughly. He agreed and conducted the necessary tests, taking samples from my body. I waited anxiously for the results, but when they arrived, nothing new was detected. Despite this, I continued to feel a sense of fear.

During this time, God reassured me by bringing to mind several Bible verses, including Joshua 1:9, which reminds us to be strong and courageous, as the Lord is always with us. I also found comfort in Isaiah 35:4, which encourages those with fearful hearts to be strong and not to fear because God will come to save us, and John 14:27, where Jesus speaks of leaving us His peace and encourages us not to let our hearts be troubled.

Though I struggled to fully trust in my faith, I reflected on how God has guided and cared for me throughout my life. I recognized the Lord as my refuge, strength, portion, deliverer, and keeper.

On another occasion, Matthew 6:34 offered me support during stressful times, reminding me not to worry about tomorrow, as each day has its own challenges. The words from Psalm 23:4 also provided me solace, as they emphasize comfort in the presence of God even in difficult situations.

One evening, I attended a dinner party, feeling uplifted by the scriptures. I was grateful for the experience and returned home with a sense of peace.

I had an appointment with my doctor a week later and arrived on time. After examining me, she referred me to another physician for further evaluation. This new doctor recommended an ultrasound and additional tests. The results came back, but nothing significant was detected. Consequently, I underwent a biopsy, and again, no clear diagnosis was made.

I returned home feeling uncertain and without any tangible results. Later, my doctor called to schedule another appointment. During this visit, she informed me that while the ultrasound and biopsy showed no conclusive findings, the overall situation was concerning, and she would be referring me to a specialist.

I faced a month of waiting to see the specialist, and during that time, fear began to overwhelm me. I found myself feeling anxious and emotional, which was difficult to manage.

3. My tears

I remember a day when I was shopping at Walmart. When the cashier rang up my items, she charged me the usual price instead of the discounted price that was advertised. Instead of expressing my disappointment with the pricing, I found myself in tears. The cashier noticed and was taken aback. She asked if I was okay and reassured me, offering to sell me the item at the discounted price. She seemed genuinely concerned and urged me to wipe my tears before completing the transaction.

There was another time at the gym when I was overwhelmed with emotions and ended up crying until my eyes were swollen. People around me became concerned and questioned me about what was happening. They suggested that I not use the gym that day but provided me with a note to show when I returned. I left feeling unsettled and terrified. In that moment, I prayed for strength, particularly given my health challenges.

One day, while sitting in my car, I found myself weeping as I recalled the prayer that Jesus made in the Garden of Gethsemane, asking, "If possible, let this cup pass from me." In that moment, I prayed tearfully, "O Lord, let this cup pass from me," aware deep down that I might have cancer. The tears seemed to flow constantly; I wept while teaching children at Sunday school and during countless moments alone in my car.

People who saw me in distress often assumed I was facing financial difficulties and offered me money, which I consistently declined. I appreciated their kindness and compassion, but my struggles were not rooted in finances. Another instance occurred when I was filling my car with gas. Suddenly, tears began streaming down my face. A man approached me, concerned, and asked if I was okay. I assured him I was fine, but he insisted that I wasn't. He mentioned wanting to see how much I was charged, a comment that confused me at the time. When I went inside to pay, I learned that he had already taken care of the bill. Upon discovering this, I cried again. In that moment, I prayed for comfort and for the grace to surrender all my worries into God's hands.

Chapter Five

I Became Sick

1. "This Is Cancer."

After anxiously waiting for a month and two weeks, the day of my appointment finally arrived, and I met the specialist doctor. My heart was racing; I did not know what to do, and I began to weep. To comfort me, my husband said, "Please, it is not cancer." I replied with certainty, "It is cancer. I didn't tell you because I knew you would be shocked if I did." "In Jesus' name," he responded, "Why don't you speak positively about your health?" I replied, "Okay, just to avoid disappointing you."

As soon as the doctor saw me, she said, "This is cancer." She did not seem to care about my emotions. At that moment, I would have been relieved if the earth had opened up and swallowed me. Immediately, she embraced both me and my husband. He looked bewildered, his facial expression betraying his worry. Though we felt helpless, I asked her in a low voice, "How can you be so sure?" She replied confidently," I have twenty-five years of experience; I know what cancer is."

I then asked, "If you can speak about it so confidently, why has it not been detected until now?" She explained, "Some types of cancer hide and cannot be easily detected. Since I began my career in this field, I have learned where it tends to hide." She continued, "I have my doubts about where it is hiding; I will need to perform a biopsy. It has gone undetected until now because the other doctors did not know which part to biopsy." I agreed to her plan and waited for the biopsy results.

The results came back in a week, and they were not pleasant; our fears were confirmed—I had cancer. The mere mention of the word "cancer" is frightening in itself. A feeling of apprehension enveloped me, as if the angel of death had arrived with all its burdens. Cancer does not discriminate; it does not care whether you are black, white, educated, or uneducated; rich, poor, a child, a youth, an adult, or elderly; married, single, beautiful, or not; plump or lean; weak or strong—anyone can be affected by it.

Since the day I received my diagnosis, many nights have been spent in tears; my sorrow felt as though it had become my sustenance. Although the doctor assured me that I had an 80% chance of survival, I struggled to accept it. A sense of unbearable gloom enveloped me, and I questioned the purpose of life, feeling that my existence had lost its meaning. Cancer can profoundly impact one's sense femininity.

2. The Cancer Card

After my examination results were delivered, I was informed that I would receive a card confirming my status as a cancer patient, essential for all subsequent actions. They explained that I would be admitted to the hospital and that my family would receive guidance on the care I would need. They mentioned that they would show me the area designated for chemotherapy. At that moment, the reality of my diagnosis hit me fully, and I felt overwhelming fear.

As I waited in line to obtain my cancer card, I was struck by the number of people around me. I found myself thinking, "Surely, not all of these individuals can be here for a cancer diagnosis." Just then, a woman from my home country approached me and said, "Only cancer patients stand in this line. In case you weren't aware." I replied, "I know. I've been told I have cancer and am here for the card." Her reaction surprised me; she expressed disbelief that someone like me, whom she described as pretty, could have cancer, and she began to cry. Her tears heightened my own anxiety, leaving me feeling even more unsettled in that moment.

As I waited in line, some of the other patients rebuked the woman who had expressed concern for me. They asked her, "Who is she to you?" I explained, "She is not related to me; she is a compatriot." This seemed to surprise them. The woman then composed herself, stating, "I will wait here until you receive your card; I cannot accept that you have cancer without seeing proof." After I was handed the card, I showed it to her. She fell silent for a moment before expressing her thoughts, saying, "May God help you; here is my number; call me. I work here. I'm sorry for alarming you! I have never seen a Habesha woman with cancer. Seeing you, a beautiful woman, facing this situation disturbed me."

I appreciated her compassion, a gesture that had a lasting impact on me.

Regarding the cancer card itself, it serves a purpose similar to that of a driver's license or a certificate awarded for completing a course. Its issuance signifies the confirmation of my cancer diagnosis. The staff explained that I must present this card every time I visit for treatment, whether at this facility or any other. The process of obtaining the card was quite difficult for me, as I struggled to accept the reality of my diagnosis until the very end. This experience also reinforced my awareness of the gravity and severity of cancer as a disease.

3. "I Will Not Undergo Chemo"

After receiving my cancer card, the medical staff informed me about the next steps, including where I would undergo chemotherapy. However, upon entering the chemotherapy area, I was overwhelmed by a sense of panic. The other patients looked different, as many were hairless and had a similar appearance, which made me feel out of place. I clung tightly to my husband and flatly refused to go any further.

Despite my husband's urging, I remained steadfast in my decision not to enter. Other newcomers, who were in the same situation, approached me and offered comfort, but eventually, it became too much for my husband, who began to cry. We both left without having gone inside.

As we drove home, I expressed my desperation, asking God to take me rather than face the drastic changes that chemotherapy would bring. That evening, I contacted a nurse to inform her of my decision not to undergo treatment. She responded firmly, explaining that refusing chemotherapy would drastically reduce my chances of survival. Despite her reminders of the potential benefits, I was filled with hopelessness and questioned the value of my existence if it meant enduring such an experience.

Later, I received a call from a woman named Eri, who had been given my phone number. She reached out to encourage me to reconsider chemotherapy, sharing her own successful recovery story. She reassured me that the side effects were temporary and sent me photos of her transformation before and after treatment. Her kindness and support provided me with some comfort, leaving me with her thoughts and prayers as the call ended.

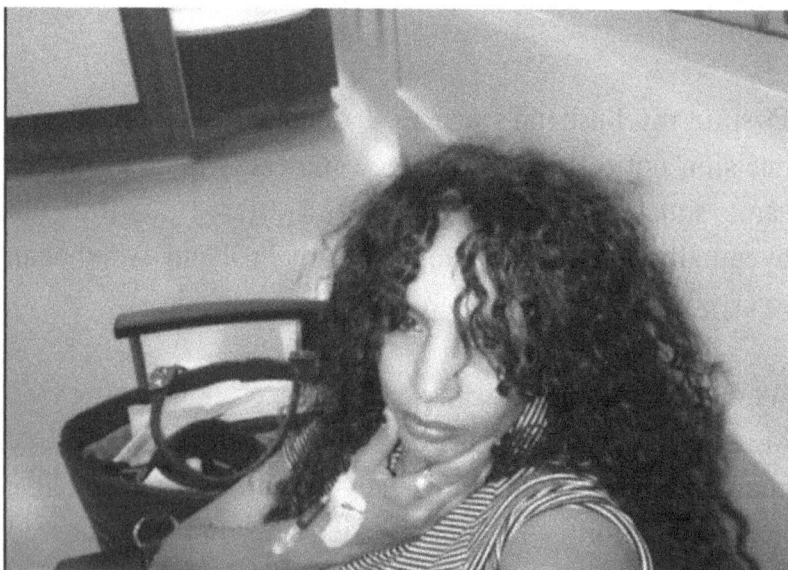

Before first chemotheraphy

After my initial decision to avoid chemotherapy, Pastor Meron reached out to me. During our conversation, I expressed my reluctance to begin treatment. He suggested that my decision lacked wisdom and shared a Bible passage with me before praying, which provided me with some support and comfort.

The following day, my doctor called to discuss my situation more urgently. She informed me of the difficulty in detecting my cancer due to its hidden nature and stressed the importance of starting chemotherapy without delay. She explained that it was crucial to address the tumor before any surgical intervention could occur. The doctor emphasized the need for treatment, detailing how even younger and older patients with severe diagnoses opted for chemotherapy to increase their chances of survival.

Faced with this information and the encouragement I had received from both Eri and Pastor Meron, I felt a shift in my perspective. I ultimately expressed my willingness to accept whatever decision was meant for me, saying, "Oh, Lord, do as you like."

Chapter Six

Its Side Effects

I do not like going to the hospital. "But now I am going to become a friend of the hospital, the doctors, and the nurses," I thought as I hesitantly approached the hospital. Upon arrival, I entered the room where I would reluctantly begin chemotherapy. The nurse assigned to me was charming and cheerful.

She took my hand and said, "My dear, I am so sorry that you are facing this illness. Hearing about cancer is heartbreaking. I need to clearly explain the side effects of chemotherapy." She continued, "The side effects can include blood disorders, nausea, vomiting, diarrhea, swelling, shortness of breath, irregular heartbeat, decreased blood pressure, fatigue, hair loss, eyebrow loss, blood clots, dry mouth, infiction in the mouth and throat irritation, mouth and throat swellings and difficulty swallowing and eyelash loss."

My heart nearly stopped, and I felt faint. "Are you okay?" she asked. "How can you expect me to be okay after sharing all this in one day?" I replied.

After a brief pause, a memory came to mind—Steven Spielberg's film featuring the alien named E.T. I remembered thinking I would look like her after finishing chemotherapy. I had watched the film as a child and recalled hiding behind my brother out of fear. When I shared this memory with the nurse, she smiled back at me.

After the doctor and nurse spoke with me, they provided books and materials containing detailed information about chemotherapy and its side effects. On my way home, I began reading the materials they had given me. As I read, I realized that I might encounter frightening situations. The thought that I could even lose my nails terrified me. The disease itself can lead a patient to lose hope, prompting thoughts like, "It would be better if I had never been born." The darkness often feels greater than the light. When everything seemed gloomy, I prayed, "Oh, my Lord, grant me your favor."

No sooner had I finished my prayer than a verse came to my heart: "The king will desire your beauty. He is your Lord; you are the most handsome of the sons of men; grace is poured upon your lips." Another verse, "No weapon formed against you shall prosper," gave me additional strength. Comforted by these words, I entered my house, singing. At that time, my greatest challenge was cancer; the trials each person faces are different, and what one person endures, another may not.

If you are facing various challenges, know that you are not alone; the Lord Jesus Christ is with you, even during your trials.

Though we encounter different tests, we must always place our hopes in God Most High alone. This truth is echoed throughout the Bible. As David the Psalmist says in Psalm 39:7, "But now, Lord, what do I look for? My hope is in you." Let us likewise place our hope in Him alone. During that very troubling time, when all seemed lost, I found the strength to lift my eyes toward Him and put my trust in Him alone.

Chapter Seven

Facing the Reality

1. "Have Your Hair Shaved!"

The day I was to begin chemotherapy finally arrived, and I found myself at the hospital compound an hour early. When my name was called and I entered the room, I was immediately struck by the somber atmosphere. My heart began to race as I took in the chemotherapy room's dim lighting and heavy mood. Just moments earlier, as I had walked through the spacious hall, my emotions overwhelmed me, and I bowed my head, tears streaming down my face as I prayed, "Lord, if it is Your will, please take this cup away from me."

The nurses tried to reassure me, but the faces around me told a different story—one of despair and anxiety. Some patients moaned softly, others wept, while a few busied themselves with magazines in an attempt to distract from their worries. Others lay flat on their backs in bed, vacant expressions on their faces. It was disheartening to see so many individuals sharing the same fate; their hairless heads marked them as kindred spirits in suffering. I thought to myself, "What awaits me is surely a reflection of their anguish." My gaze fell on a woman with missing toenails, and fear gripped me even tighter.

Noticing my distress, the nurses urged me to move forward, saying, "We don't have time; you need to start your treatment." I replied, "Please, give me just a moment." As I began to count slowly—one, two—my hesitation seemed to test their patience. Finally, one nurse suggested, "The hospital has a chapel. Would you like to go there and pray? There's a priest who can help." I shook my head, dismissing the offer. In that moment, all the promises I had held onto seemed to fade away. Feeling profoundly aggrieved, I burst into tears.

As I wept, the words of King David echoed in my mind: "My tears have been my food day and night, while people say to me all day long, 'Where is your God?'"

Like David, my tears felt like my only sustenance. The other patients in the hospital seemed like strangers to me, individuals from another world. Since my arrival, I could sense their astonishment when they looked at me, as if they were saying, "It is her first time." My long, curly hair set me apart in that environment; I was the only one among them with hair. After some time, a nurse commented, "Your hair is very beautiful. When you come back for your next appointment, consider shaving it to spare yourself the pain."

A fellow cancer patient added, "I had my hair cut before starting chemo; it's a good idea to shave it off beforehand." I nodded in agreement. Another nurse suggested, "Cut your hair and donate it to a cancer society." Again, I agreed. Their admiration for my hair made me realize I had taken it for granted, and in that moment, I understood the significance that hair holds for many women.

After I had my hair cut and completed my first round of chemotherapy, I noticed that my hair had not changed at all. A woman voiced her frustration, asking, "Why did you have your hair cut? Wouldn't it have been better for you to see what would happen to it?" I responded, "Alright, I won't shave it. I'll wait and see if my hair falls out."

2. I Gave in to My Daughter's Idea

After my second round of chemotherapy, I returned home and, while lying in bed that evening, I noticed a significant amount of hair on my pillow. When I touched my hair, it simply fell out. The following day, a friend suggested, "Let me take you to a hair salon so you can have your hair shaved and buy a wig." I struggled to accept this reality and replied, "I will not do it." At that point, I had developed bald patches on my head.

When my daughter came home from school, I saw the shock in her eyes. Suppressing her feelings, she said, "Let me go with you to a hair salon. Let's shave your hair and buy a wig." Eventually, I agreed, and together we went to a hair shop where I had my hair shaved. However, we disagreed on which wig to purchase. She wanted me to buy a wig that matched the length of my lost hair, while I preferred a shorter one. In the end, I decided to go along with her preference. She was pleased, and I bought a long wig and tried it on.

As I looked in the mirror, I noticed how different I appeared, and I found it challenging to accept this new look. A question arose within me: "Will I be able to get used to it?"

3. The Challenge Continued

I did not find the third round of chemotherapy to be very painful, but I did lose all my eyebrows, and my nails began to darken. By the fourth round, I noticed significant changes in my skin and overall appearance. I lost all the hair on my body, and my eyebrows and eyelashes disappeared completely. When my nails fell off, I felt like I resembled an alien woman from another world, much like the other women I had seen before me. After the fifth round, I received treatment to determine whether the tumor was still present.

When the tumor showed no change, a high dose of chemotherapy was prescribed, and I began that treatment. My body underwent drastic changes, and I felt like a completely different woman. Looking in the mirror, I was shocked by how I appeared; I hardly looked human. My husband offered words of encouragement, saying, "There is no one as beautiful as you," but I found it challenging to accept. As I navigated these changes, it became absolutely necessary for me to prepare for the sixth round of chemotherapy.

When I underwent this round of chemotherapy, I became very weak and struggled with everyday tasks; I could neither lift things nor take a bath. As a result, I lost interest in meeting people. I realized that individuals with cancer often prefer to avoid social interactions because comments and questions from others can be as painful as the illness itself. Additionally, my swollen tongue made eating a challenging experience. I found it difficult to move from one place to another, further isolating me during this difficult time.

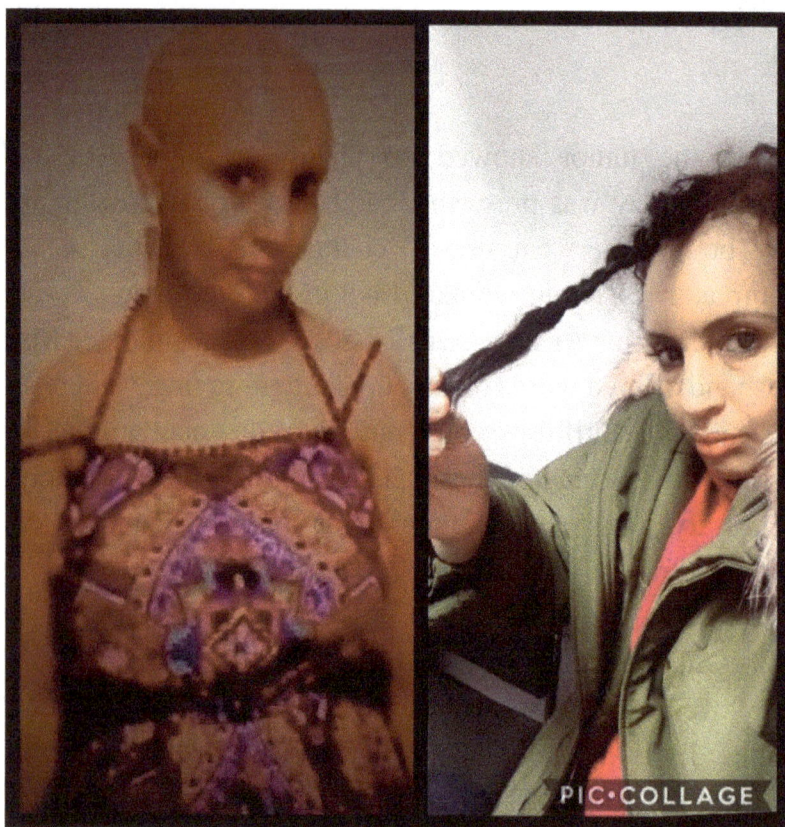

Before and after

4. I Was Visited By His Presence

One day, I found myself consumed by bitterness and cried out to my Lord, "What kind of sin have I committed that all of this is happening to me? Are you not my father, even if I have made mistakes? Will you not have mercy on me?" In the midst of this turmoil, a passage came to my heart.

It was a response reminiscent of the words from the book of Ezekiel: "He asked me, 'Son of man, can these bones live?' I replied, 'Sovereign Lord, you alone know.' Then he said to me, 'Prophesy to these bones and say to them, "Dry bones, hear the word of the Lord! This is what the Sovereign Lord says to these bones: I will make breath enter you, and you will come to life. I will attach tendons to you and make flesh come upon you, and cover you with skin; I will put breath in you, and you will come to life.

Then you will know that I am the Lord."' So I prophesied as I was commanded. And as I was prophesying, there was a noise, a rattling sound, and the bones came together, bone to bone. He continued, 'Son of man, these bones are the people of Israel. They say, "Our bones are dried up and our hope is gone; we are cut off." Therefore, prophesy and say to them: "This is what the Sovereign Lord says:

My people, I am going to open your graves. Then you, my people, will know that I am the Lord, when I bring you up from your graves. I will put my Spirit in you and you will live and settle you in your own land. Then you will know that I, the Lord, have spoken, and I have done it," declares the Lord."' (Ezekiel 37:1-14).

As I reflected on this passage, I found a sense of hope amidst my struggles, a reminder that there is power in words and the promise of restoration.

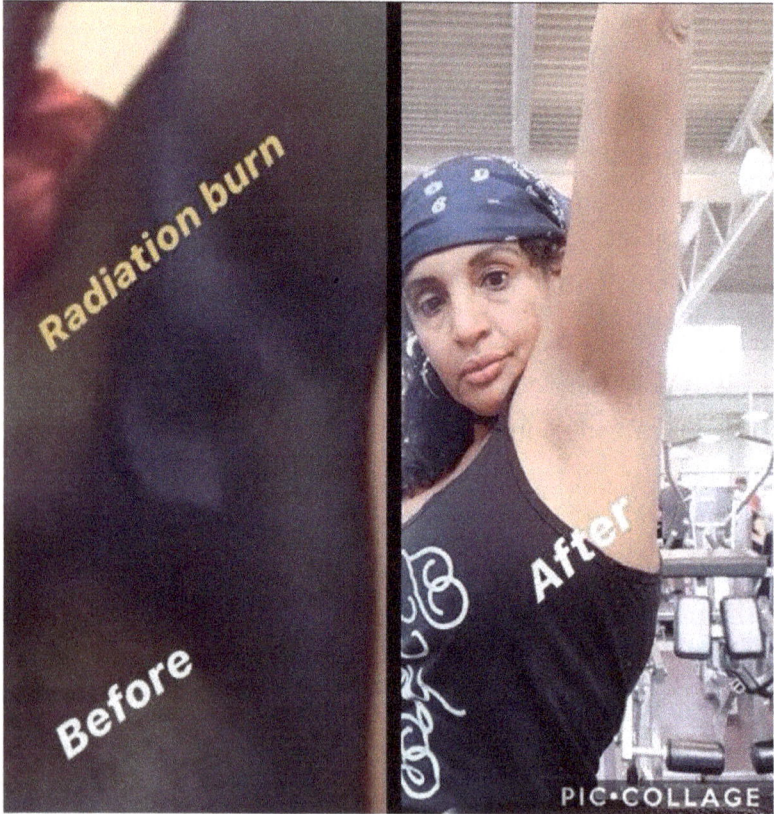

Right after reading the passage from Ezekiel, I experienced a powerful movement of the Holy Spirit within me. The presence of God took hold of my entire being, bringing a profound sense of comfort and hope. Despite the physical changes I had undergone, including the loss of my hair and beauty, I sensed that restoration was possible. This understanding eased my feelings of hopelessness, and I felt enveloped in His love, protection, and care, which brought me a deep sense of peace.

I prayed earnestly, expressing my gratitude: "Thank you, Lord, for the promise of restoration. I have faith that you will rejuvenate my body and bring back my former beauty. I trust in you to transform this physical state and grant me life anew." No matter how daunting my circumstances became, I committed to staying strong and maintaining a positive outlook.

While I had no control over cancer, I knew that it could not diminish my faith or my perspective on life. I resolved to keep fighting until I no longer could, much like David's plea in Psalms 31:1: "In you, LORD, I have taken refuge; let me never be put to shame; deliver me in your righteousness."

Later, I felt led to read Ezekiel 47. After that reading, I turned my heart to prayer once more, saying, "Lord, I desire a deeper knowledge of you and a closer relationship with you. I long to love with a profound love; please, let me overflow with your Spirit as you did for Ezekiel."

In these moments, I remained hopeful and steadfast in my faith journey.

Another time, the Holy Spirit guided me to read Ezekiel 47. After reading, I prayed, "Oh, Lord! I want to get to know You. I desire to have a close fellowship with You and to love with a deep love. Oh, Lord, cause me to overflow with Your Spirit as You did for Ezekiel.

Jesus, I want to worship You and You alone. You are my Lord, my God, my King; You are worthy of all my worship. Bind my heart with Yours. Whatever comes my way in life, I need Your power, grace, and love. I want to respond to every situation in a manner that glorifies You. I long to draw very close to You. May Your Spirit emanate from within me in everything I do and say. I want my mind, my strength, and my heart to be focused not on myself or my circumstances, but on You, Jesus. I want You and You alone."

Then I was comforted; I was filled with the Holy Spirit overflowing. The Holy Spirit filled my bedroom, and I felt the presence of a Spirit I could not control and take hold of my entire being. I said, "Jesus, I love You. You are with me."

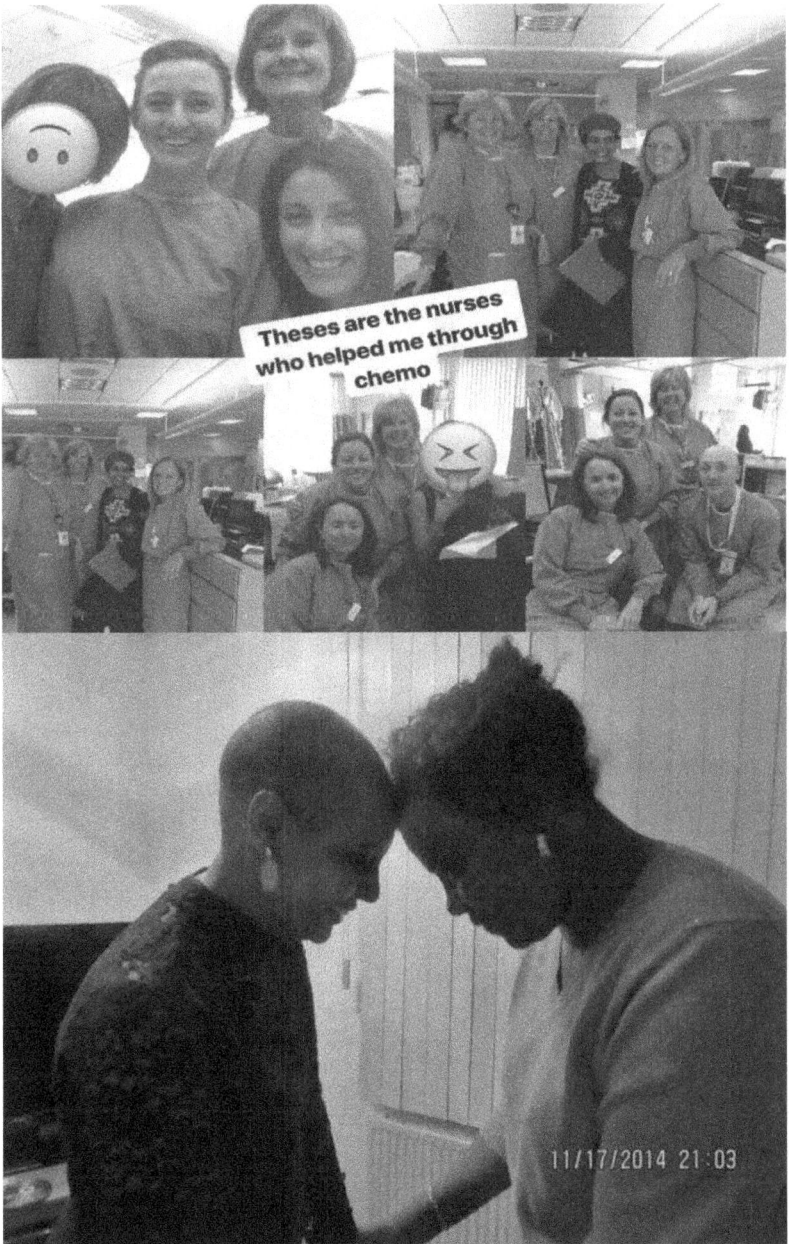

Theses are the nurses who helped me through chemo

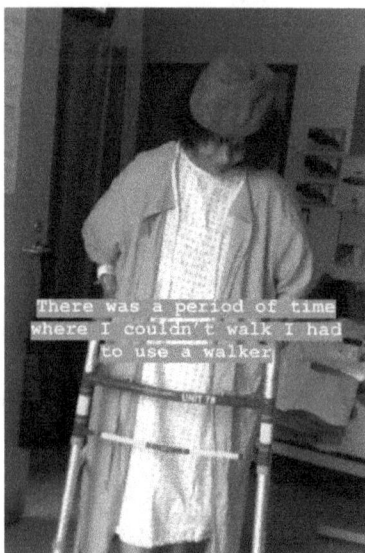

There was a period of time where I couldn't walk I had to use a walker

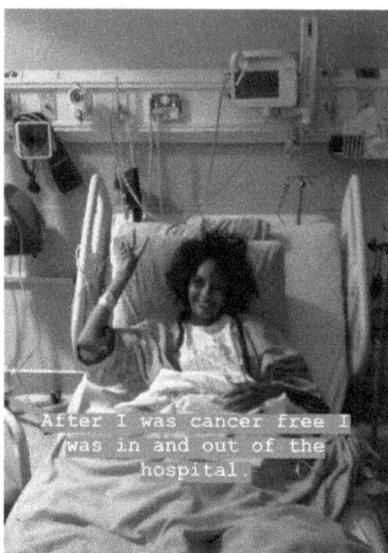

After I was cancer free I was in and out of the hospital.

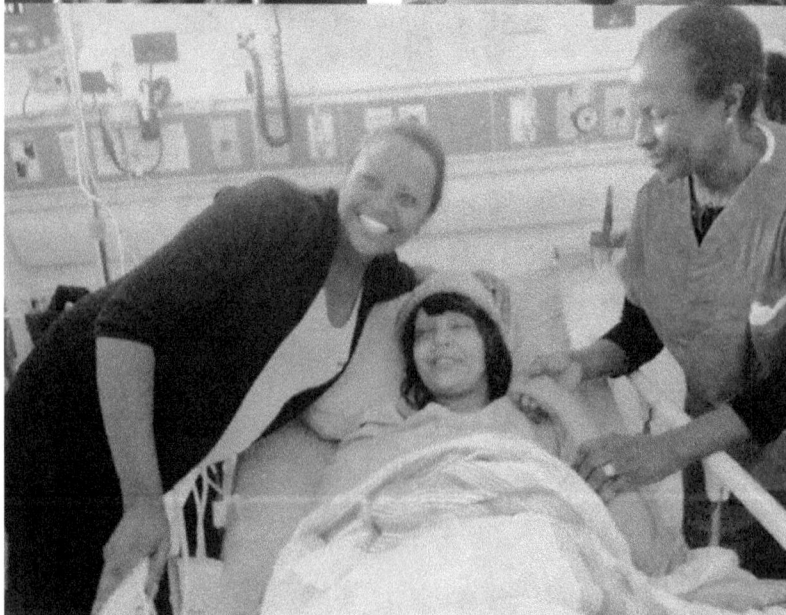

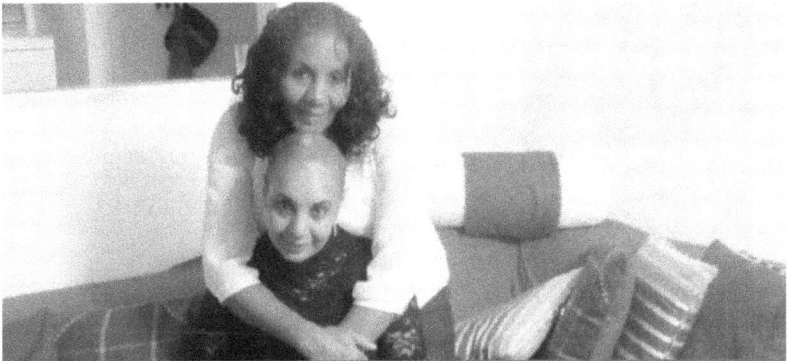

Dear n doctor and nurses thanks to each one of you .I am humbled and thrilled to be alive, and am so excited for this honor. I do not take it lightly and will do anything to glorify God. You all have no idea what this means to me. You're hard work does not go unnoticed thank you for being so compassionate

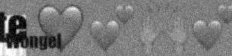

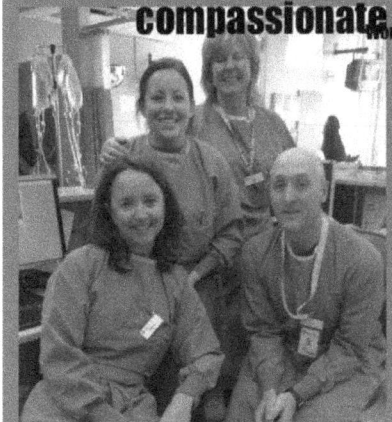

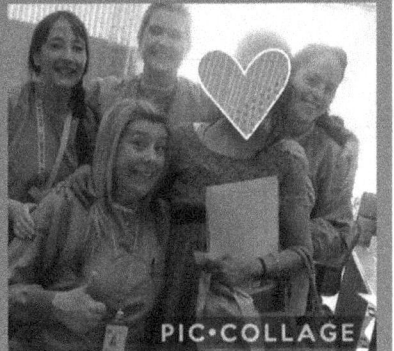

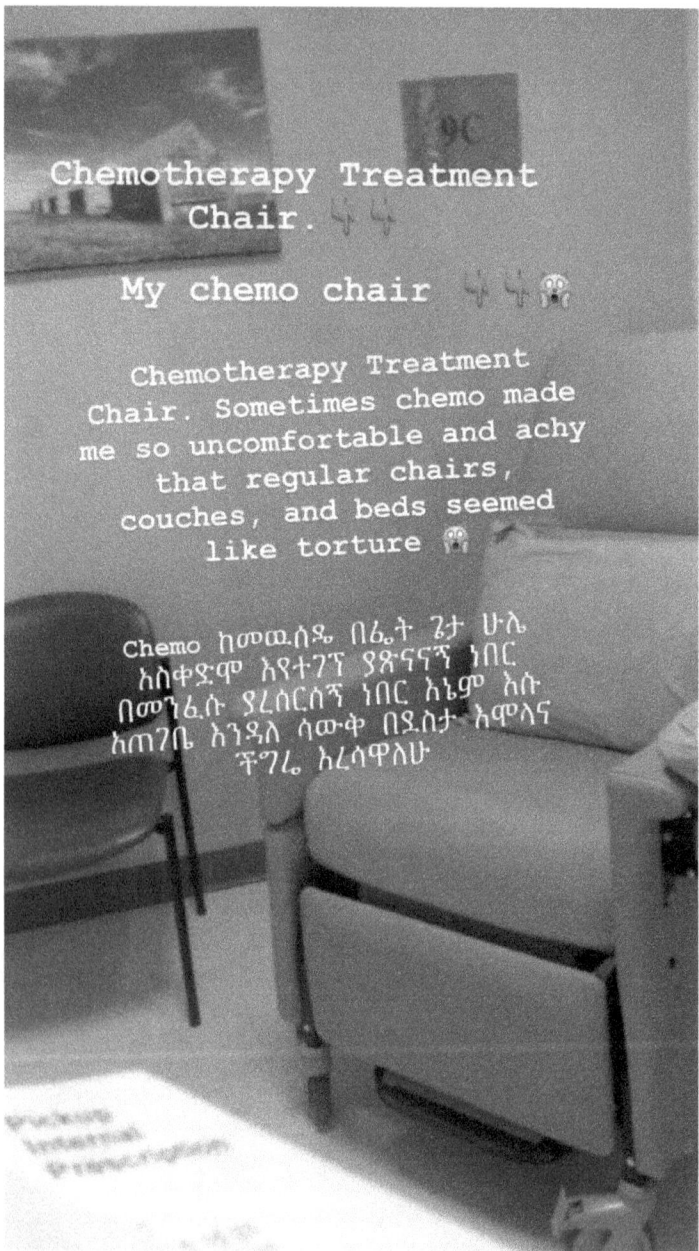

Chemotherapy Treatment Chair. 🪑🪑

My chemo chair 🪑🪑😰

Chemotherapy Treatment Chair. Sometimes chemo made me so uncomfortable and achy that regular chairs, couches, and beds seemed like torture 😰

Chemo ከመዉሰዴ በፊት ጊታ ሁሌ አስቀድሞ እየተገፕ ያጸናናኝ ነበር በመንፈሱ ያረሰርሰኝ ነበር እኔም እሱ አጠገቤ እንዳለ ሳውቅ በደስታ እሞላና ቸግሬ አረሳዋለሁ

Chapter Eight

I Experienced Remarkable Healing

Despite the challenges I faced, I found comfort in the presence of the Holy Spirit. Yet, I felt the ongoing struggle of spiritual warfare. I longed to worship my Lord with outstretched arms, but pain often held me back. I wanted to express my emotions through tears in His presence, but fear of marrying my face from the effects of chemotherapy kept me from doing so. My tongue was swollen from medication intended to reduce its size, which affected my enjoyment of food. Remarkably, all these physical afflictions arose just three days after I had encountered the overwhelming presence of the Holy Ghost in my life.

During this difficult time, I lost hope in my fight against cancer. Daily coping with the disease was exhausting and frightening, leaving me to question, "When will I find rest?"

Confusion took hold of me, and I wept, articulating my struggle: "God is with me; but why is all this happening? I find it hard to worship You." In the midst of this turmoil, I randomly opened my Bible, and it fell open to Judges 6:13, which reads, "But if the Lord is with us, why has all this happened to us? Where are all His wonders that our ancestors told us about when they said, 'Did not the Lord bring us up out of Egypt?' But now the Lord has abandoned us and given us into the hand of Midian." In that moment, I called out, "Jesus Christ, where is Your power? Where is Your miraculous work? Where is Your healing? Are You with me?"

I prayed before the Lord, saying, "Forgive me for all the sins I have committed; please help me; remember me in Your mercy; glorify Your name. I am not ashamed of You; I know Your name heals me, and I have no doubt that You will completely remove this disease from me. You are great; Your hand that did wonders in the past does the same today."

I found comfort in the words of God in 2 Corinthians 12:9–10: "But he said to me, 'My grace is sufficient for you, for my power is made perfect in weakness.' Therefore I will boast all the more gladly about my weaknesses, so that Christ's power may rest on me. That is why, for Christ's sake, I delight in weaknesses, in insults, in hardships, in persecutions, in difficulties. For when I am weak, then I am strong." Additionally, I meditated on Psalm 118:17, reminding myself that I would not die, but live. During this period, I was blessed by the spiritual songs of Kalkidan (Lili) Tilahun, which I listened to repeatedly.

One important lesson I learned is that during such challenging times, Satan seeks to embitter us toward God and lead us away from our Lord Jesus Christ, rather than encouraging us to worship Him.

Life can unexpectedly shift us from one situation to another in the blink of an eye due to unforeseen sad events. However, regardless of what happens, God remains with us. When we turn our eyes toward Him, peace comes, and we need not be afraid. We should lift our eyes to Him, focus on His mercy and kindness, and trust in Him.

The verse "For the Mighty One has done great things for me; holy is His name" (Luke 1:49) resonates deeply with my experience. After undergoing 13 surgeries and 6 rounds of chemotherapy and radiation therapy, I faced significant challenges, including a severe burn on half of my body, leading to fears that I might live with these effects indefinitely. I did not expect my body to return to its former state as it had deteriorated significantly.

However, after enduring this ordeal, I experienced remarkable healing through my faith in Jesus Christ. I found strength and resilience in my journey. I want to remind others grappling with cancer that they are not alone, no matter how difficult the struggle may seem. God remains a source of support and hope.

To those who are enduring suffering and hardship, remember that you are not alone. The Lord who healed me can also bring healing to you. As it says in Psalm 34:19, "The righteous person may have many troubles, but the Lord delivers him from them all." Though I faced significant challenges with my physical health due to

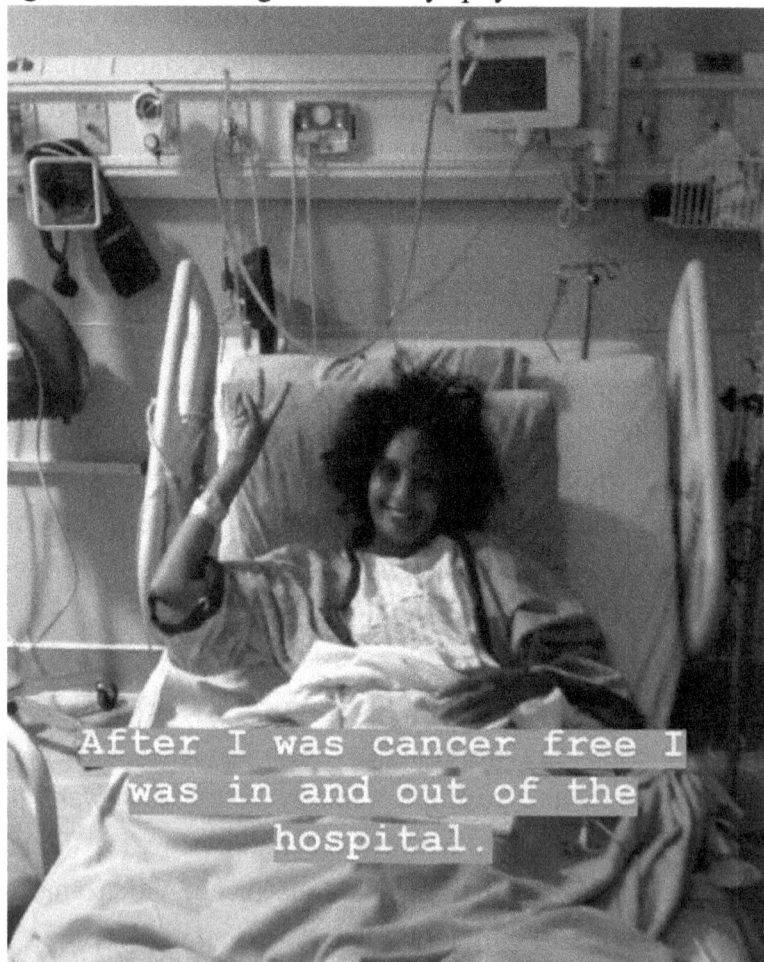

After I was cancer free I was in and out of the hospital.

surgeries, chemotherapy, and radiation, my spirit remained untouched by negativity.

The Scriptures provide reassurance in 2 Corinthians 4:16-18: "Therefore we do not lose heart. Though outwardly we are wasting away, yet inwardly we are being renewed day by day. For our light and momentary troubles are achieving for us an eternal glory that far outweighs them all. So we fix our eyes not on what is seen, but on what is unseen, since what is seen is temporary, but what is unseen is eternal." Praise be to God, who will never abandon us in our times of need.

Chapter Nine

A Believer Will Never Get Sick

1. The minister condemned her

During the days I was confined to bed with cancer, I began to hear things I never thought I would. I could hardly believe my ears when a preacher said, "People who get sick are sinners—those who have sinned greatly." Hearing such a thing struck me deeply.

I remembered a kind and loving sister who used to visit patients in hospitals and feed the hungry. She suddenly fell ill, just before I received my own cancer diagnosis. Until then, she had never been sick. The doctors informed her that she had only three months left to live. The news left her in shock, prompting her to reach out to various ministers for support.

One day, she called me, tears in her voice, to share her experience: "A minister came to see me and said, 'Confess all the sins you've committed. What has happened to you is the result of not attending church and prioritizing money over God.'" His words made her already difficult situation even worse.

I felt a surge of anger at the minister's insensitivity. I said, "Please give me his phone number. I want to talk to him." She replied sadly, "Wongel, please let it go. If he wants to judge me or curse me, that's on him. I'm in God's hands now.

Wongel This preacher is judging me without knowing anything about my circumstances. The reason I can't attend church every Sunday is that I have to work hard to make the monthly mortgage payments on my home and to provide a better life for my children. I am not backsliding; I pray every day and help anyone in need. I have confessed all my sins, yet I am left wondering what special sin I might have committed that no one else has.

A question arose within me: "This woman has been told she will die in three months; how do we condemn her instead of offering comfort?"

I said to her, "Cheer up; this too shall pass. You are not sick because of sin. We are all sinners. Everyone goes through difficult times not necessarily because of their sins. God is not human; He does not judge us or inflict illness upon us as punishment for sin. Look at the disciples of Jesus Christ; they endured tribulations as well. This preacher's teaching is not biblical."

I shared some Bible passages for her to read and tried to comfort her by saying, "Some suffering is simply a temptation from Satan, as seen in Job 1:1-2. Focus your eyes on the Lord and don't listen to unbiblical advice from some ministers. Besides, you know where you will go if you die now."

This sister has passed away, and the Lord has called her home. Her funeral attracted a large number of attendees and was broadcast live on social media, allowing many to express their condolences. Her impact was evident in the way people shared their problems with her, highlighting her compassion and kindness.

Although she was not a preacher, singer, or actively involved in formal church ministry, she touched the hearts of many through her love ,kindness and support. Her legacy serves as a reminder that one can have a profound influence on others through genuine care and connection, regardless of their official role in a religious community.

2. Hidden Sins

Seven years after this my friend passed away, I found myself facing a cancer diagnosis—something I had never anticipated. In the wake of my diagnosis, I grappled with a troubling question: Was this illness a consequence of some hidden sin in my life? I firmly believe the answer is no. While I acknowledge my imperfections, I understand that developing cancer is not directly tied to specific sins or a lack of closeness to God.

Nevertheless, I encountered various reactions from those around me. Some urged me to confess any hidden sins, while others prayed for divine mercy on my behalf. A few suggested that my illness stemmed from a lack of faith, and others advised that I apologize to anyone I might have wronged. There were individuals who viewed themselves as more righteous, believing that my cancer was a result of my sins. In those moments, as they prayed for my forgiveness, I found myself silently praying for them.

When visiting the sick, it is important to avoid adding to their anxiety and suffering. People experience different hardships; some face significant struggles while others seem to succeed across various aspects of life. It is not biblical to conclude that success equates to righteousness or that suffering is a direct result of sin. We cannot fully understand how God works. He does not operate on a principle of punishment for every misstep, nor does He afflict individuals with disease solely because of sin.

The story of Job in the Bible serves as a poignant example. He endured significant trials not as a punishment for sin but as part of a broader divine purpose. While God can indeed hold individuals accountable for their actions, it is important to recognize that not every challenge or hardship is linked to sin.

Some people believe that only those who are wicked suffer, suggesting that God is on the side of the righteous and will remove their troubles. However, it is important to recognize that suffering is not limited to the wicked. This idea aligns with the perspective of Job's friends, as seen in Job 4:7-9. We should avoid concluding that we are facing difficulties because we have sinned. Instead, suffering may provide an opportunity to demonstrate our commitment to God.

When visiting the sick, if no particular words come to mind to share at that moment, it may be more appropriate to remain silent rather than attributing their illness to Satan, a lack of faith, or personal sin. It is beneficial to refrain from making unnecessary remarks. During my own illness, I encountered comments from various individuals and ministers suggesting that I confess any hidden sins or attributing my troubles to a lack of faith.

It is a common belief that only the wicked suffer, but this perspective can be misleading. We should be cautious not to assume that difficulties or suffering are always linked to personal wrongdoing. While it is true that God may discipline believers for sin, we should avoid making judgments based on limited understanding. Suffering can sometimes serve as an opportunity to affirm our commitment to God.

During one of my days as a cancer patient, a woman I barely knew called me after hearing about my diagnosis. She said, "I had cancer four years ago. Be strong; nothing will happen to you. Just pray earnestly." However, this woman, who sought to comfort me, later became ill and was hospitalized. There, doctors informed her that her cancer had returned and spread throughout her body, giving her just 2 months to live.

This woman had a deep love and respect for the Lord. When I learned of her situation, I reached out to offer comfort, but she instead comforted me. She stated with conviction, "I will not die, but live." Despite her worsening condition, she continued to praise the Lord. During one of our conversations, she tearfully shared that a minister had advised her, "Confess if you have committed any sin." Additionally, another person told her, "A Christian never gets sick; all diseases are from Satan."

I advised her, "Do not listen to what people say; focus on what the Word says. Do not base your faith on their comments." Unfortunately, this sister is no longer with us;

the Lord called her home. After her passing, another individual attempted to console me by saying, "She died because she had very little faith. If she had the same faith as you, she would have recovered."

I do not understand why the Lord spared my life while taking hers. It is not a matter of differing faith levels; God has His reasons for all that He does. As it is said, "And the God of all grace, who called you to his eternal glory in Christ, after you have suffered a little while, will himself restore you and make you strong, firm, and steadfast. To him be the power forever and ever. Amen."

It's important to recognize that we should not hastily conclude that personal suffering is a punishment for sin. While it is true that God may discipline us for our wrongdoings, suffering can also serve as an opportunity to demonstrate our commitment and faithfulness to Him.

When visiting the sick or those in distress, it's crucial to approach the situation with sensitivity. If we do not have the right words of encouragement or understanding to share, it is often wiser to remain silent than to make assumptions about their condition.

Statements such as "It is Satan that caused this disease" or "You are suffering due to a lack of faith" can be harmful and unhelpful.

Your experience exemplifies this, as you encountered various responses during your own illness, including calls to confess hidden sins or to reassess your faith. These reactions can add unnecessary pressure during an already challenging time.

Ultimately, our understanding of suffering should lead us to compassion rather than judgment. Instead of speculating on the reasons for someone else's struggles, we can focus on providing support and encouragement, recognizing that suffering is a complex part of the human experience that can strengthen one's commitment to God.

Some people believe that only the wicked suffer, maintaining that God supports the righteous and will ultimately remove their troubles. However, we must understand that suffering is not limited to those who are wicked. This viewpoint aligns with the perspective of Job's friends (Job 4:7-9). We should refrain from concluding that we are facing difficulties solely because of our sins. Sometimes, suffering provides us with an opportunity to demonstrate our commitment to God.

When visiting the sick, if we find ourselves without a specific message to share, it may be more appropriate to remain silent rather than attributing their illness to a lack of faith or sin. We should avoid making unnecessary statements. During my own experience with illness, I encountered various individuals and ministers who suggested, "Confess your sins, particularly the hidden ones; you are facing challenges because of your lack of faith."

It is a common misconception that suffering only affects the wicked. As we learn from the story of Job, not all suffering is a direct result of personal wrongdoing. While it is true that God may discipline us for our sins, it is important not to judge others based on our limited understanding. Suffering can indeed serve as an opportunity to reaffirm our commitment to God.

Suffering is a universal experience that affects individuals across various circumstances and backgrounds. It is important to understand that suffering is not always a direct punishment for sin. Many factors can contribute to human suffering, including natural events, illness, and life's inherent challenges. This perspective encourages compassion and empathy, enabling us to support one another rather than making assumptions about the reasons behind someone else's struggles. Recognizing that suffering is a shared aspect of the human experience can foster a deeper understanding of the complexities of life and promote a more supportive community.

1 Peter 1:6-7 emphasizes the idea that experiencing trials and challenges can lead to spiritual growth and the strengthening of one's faith. The passage reflects on how, even in the midst of grief caused by various difficulties, believers can find reasons to rejoice due to the assurance of their faith's genuineness. The verse compares the testing of faith to the refining process of gold, suggesting that while gold can perish, faith that is tested can result in praise, honor, and glory at the revelation of Jesus Christ. This teaching encourages the belief that trials can ultimately serve a meaningful purpose in the development of one's faith.

3. Trusting in the All-Knowing GOD

There was a sister who dedicated herself to serving the church, with her husband as the worship team leader. Together, they had four children, all of whom actively participated in church ministry. When she became seriously ill and went to the hospital, she was diagnosed with stage four cancer. After a month and two weeks, she passed away, leaving behind her husband and children. Is it appropriate to conclude, "The Lord took this woman home because she sinned"? Many devoted individuals have experienced serious illnesses and have ultimately gone home to the Lord when their time came. It is not just to assume that God's wrath was upon them.

Consider the case of Kathryn Kuhlman, a woman God used significantly in ministry. She served faithfully and loved the Lord, healing many people through her work. Despite the amazing miracles achieved through her, she was not healed from the cancer she faced. Similarly, Pastor Myles Munroe died alongside his wife while on a mission to spread the word. He had devoted his life to serving others, yet he, along with ten other ministers and some of their spouses, tragically perished in a plane crash in Cuba on May 21, 2018. It would be misguided to conclude that "all these individuals died because they had committed sin."

When faced with situations we do not fully understand, it is essential to refrain from making assumptions. Instead of hastily judging or speaking without knowledge, we should approach these matters with prayer, waiting for the Lord's will regarding those who are experiencing challenges. It is vital to recognize that we should not be quick to pass judgment on circumstances we do not fully grasp; rather, we should trust in the wisdom of the All-Knowing GOD

Chapter Ten

Why Did We Go Through Hardship

"Not only so, but we also glory in our sufferings, because we know that suffering produces perseverance; perseverance, character; and character, hope. And hope does not put us to shame, because God's love has been poured out into our hearts through the Holy Spirit, who has been given to us." – Romans 5:3-5.

I have come to understand the importance of patience through my suffering. The challenges I've faced have deepened my faith in the Lord. The apostle James, in his epistle, advises us: "Consider it pure joy, my brothers and sisters, whenever you face trials of many kinds, because you know that the testing of your faith produces perseverance." – James 1:2-3.

When confronted with trials, it's essential to look beyond the immediate difficulties. We should hold onto the belief that God will guide us through these times. We must trust that after this period of darkness, a new dawn will break.

God allows us to endure suffering and hardship so that we might serve as witnesses, inspiring others to change and praise Him after hearing our testimonies. When Joseph encountered his brothers many years after they sold him, he said, "You intended to harm me, but God intended it for good to accomplish what is now being done, the saving of many lives" (Genesis 50:20). During my own challenging times, I often heard comforting voices asking, "Have you gone through all this?" By fixing my eyes on the Lord and leaning on Him throughout my suffering, I was able to navigate that darkness. This journey has instilled in me a deeper sense of humility.

In relation to suffering, the apostle Paul offers insight into his experiences: "Are they servants of Christ? (I am out of my mind to talk like this.) I am more. I have worked much harder, been in prison more frequently, been flogged more severely, and been exposed to death again and again. Five times I received from the Jews the forty lashes minus one.

Three times I was beaten with rods, once I was pelted with stones, three times I was shipwrecked, I spent a night and a day in the open sea. I have been constantly on the move. I have been in danger from rivers, in danger from bandits, in danger from my fellow Jews, in danger from Gentiles; in danger in the city, in danger in the country, in danger at sea; and in danger from false believers. I have labored and toiled and have often gone without sleep; I have known hunger and thirst and have often gone without food; I have been cold and naked. Besides everything else, I face daily the pressure of my concern for all the churches" (2 Corinthians 11:23-29; see also 2 Timothy 3:10-12; 1 Peter 4:12-16; Hebrews 11:16-33; 1 Thessalonians 3:2-4; Acts 14:22; and John 16:33).

The apostle Paul's experiences illustrate that he faced a wide array of trials and challenges throughout his life, despite his devotion to the Lord. His suffering was not a result of sin or a lack of faith; rather, it reflects the reality of life on Earth. Similarly, Jesus endured suffering, as did many of His followers. It is important to recognize that while different individuals may face varying forms of suffering, hardship is a shared aspect of the human experience.

There is a prevalent belief among some preachers that suggests righteous individuals will not suffer, instead receiving continuous blessings. However, Scripture indicates that all Christians will encounter tribulation at some point in their lives.

In a conversation, a woman expressed her confusion regarding the difficulties she faced, questioning if they stemmed from her character. After relaying a response from a preacher who attributed her struggles to a lack of fasting, praying, or church attendance, she sought clarity. I

119

reassured her that suffering is an unavoidable part of life for everyone. It is crucial to discern that hardships do not necessarily indicate a person's moral standing or spiritual practice. Instead, they serve as a reminder that even the Lord and His followers faced challenges during their lives. It is essential to find comfort in this truth rather than in the opinions of others.

Hardships can often feel overwhelming and seemingly endless, but it is important to remember that there will come a time when relief will be granted. In moments of suffering, some individuals may offer their own interpretations of the challenges one faces, suggesting that they stem from personal failings or hidden sins. However, it is crucial to understand that having faith in a compassionate and unwavering God can provide comfort and strength during difficult times.

When encountering various trials, it can be beneficial to humbly seek strength and grace from the Lord, asking for support to endure the challenges faced. Encouragement and support from those around us—be it friends, family, or members of the faith community—can also play a significant role in helping individuals navigate their suffering. Positive reinforcement such as "be strong" or "cheer up" can provide much-needed hope without adding to one's burdens. In situations of distress, the presence of supportive individuals, like pastors or friends, can provide comfort through prayer, encouragement, and the sharing of uplifting messages.

In times of tribulation, it can be beneficial to practice self-encouragement and draw strength from one's faith. The example of David in 1 Samuel 30:6 illustrates the importance of finding strength within oneself and relying on God during challenging moments. Instead of becoming overwhelmed by external circumstances or the opinions of others, it is essential to take the initiative to uplift oneself.

Encouraging oneself can mean recognizing personal resilience and taking the time to acknowledge one's efforts and progress. While seeking support from others can be valuable, there are times when turning inward and reaffirming one's trust in God's power and strength is necessary. This self-encouragement can help to foster a sense of hope and perseverance when faced with adversity.

The Bible features several figures who exemplify the concept of self-encouragement through their faith and actions. Here are a few notable examples:

1. David: As mentioned in 1 Samuel 30:6, David encouraged himself in the Lord when faced with adversity, particularly during the time when his followers were

threatening to harm him. He turned to God for strength and guidance.

2. Paul: The Apostle Paul frequently wrote about the importance of perseverance and self-encouragement in his letters. In 2 Corinthians 1:8-10, he reflects on suffering and the comfort he finds in God, emphasizing the importance of relying on divine strength during difficult times.

3. Job: Despite his immense suffering and loss, Job maintained his faith and continued to seek God. His dialogues in the book of Job reveal a struggle yet a commitment to trust in God's plan, showcasing a form of self-encouragement as he affirms his belief in God's justice and sovereignty.

4. Moses: In the face of significant challenges while leading the Israelites, Moses often sought encouragement from God. For instance, in Exodus 14, during the Israelites' escape from Egypt, he reminded them to "be still" and trust in God's deliverance.

5. Nehemiah: When faced with opposition while rebuilding the walls of Jerusalem, Nehemiah encouraged himself and the people by reminding them of God's greatness and the importance of their work (Nehemiah 4:14).

These figures illustrate that self-encouragement often involves a combination of inner strength, reliance on faith, and affirming one's purpose and identity, even in the face of challenges.

Chapter Eleven

Being Yourself

Most of the time, our compatriots do not talk about their problems; they only reflect their happiness. As a result, we may think that others are doing well in life while we are facing various trials. I remember a woman I knew who often compared herself to others and complained to God. She said to me, "My car has broken down; they have two cars. It has been a long time since I arrived in this country, while they just came recently. Yet, look, everything is going well for them. Have you seen so-and-so's marriage? They love each other so much, while you know my marriage situation."

I replied, "Most of the time, our compatriots do not discuss their problems. We are reluctant to share what we are going through or what has happened to us, which may lead others to idealize our lives. Many people complain bitterly to God; however, we should avoid comparing ourselves to others. Remember, there is always someone who seems greater than us—whether in education, beauty, wealth, or other aspects."

I continued, "What you should focus on is being more like Jesus in your everyday life. The more time you spend with

125

Him, the more you will reflect His character. You will find yourself thirsting for Him and talking about Him; when you do, you won't concern yourself as much with what others are doing. You will learn to be content with what you have, saying, 'I have Jesus; what else do I want?' You will begin to lean on the Lord. Additionally, it is important to praise Him for everything you have been given. Be thankful in all circumstances, and remember to thank the Lord even for what has not yet been done for you."

As for me, I do not compare myself to others; I have achieved nothing by doing so. What I gained instead was a tendency to complain bitterly to God. I have no jealousy or envy; the only thing that truly amazes me is my Lord Jesus Christ. It has been a long time since I gave up such complaints prompted by comparisons with others. I realized early on that to maintain my peace, I should focus on my own life rather than measure it against that of others. Instead of comparing myself to others, I choose to focus on what the Lord has given me and express my gratitude.

I thank my Lord for everything I have, no matter how big or small. I have learned to replace complaints with gratitude. Nowadays, I genuinely feel happiness when I see someone else with more or living more comfortably than I do. I even pray that God may bless them abundantly. I no longer compare myself with anyone else. As stated in our

Bible in 1Thessalonians 5:18, "Give thanks in all circumstances; for this is the will of God for you in Christ Jesus."

When we start thanking the Lord in all circumstances, we may see positive changes. Comparing ourselves to others allows Satan to take advantage of our thoughts and rob us of joy and peace. The Bible reminds us in Galatians 6:4-5, "Each of you must examine your own actions. Then you can take pride in yourself alone, without comparing yourself to someone else."

Another passage states, "We wouldn't dare to class ourselves or compare ourselves with those who commend themselves. When they measure themselves by themselves and compare themselves to themselves, they are not wise" (2 Corinthians 10:12).

It's important to recognize the significance of focusing on our own journey rather than comparing ourselves to others. Each individual is uniquely created by God, and we all have distinct purposes and paths to follow. As stated in Jeremiah 29:11, God has plans for each of us that are meant to bring hope and a positive future.

Through challenges and suffering, it's natural for others to express concern, asking when things will improve.

127

However, we can find comfort in the belief that God remains faithful, and that even in difficult times, there is the promise of eventual healing and prosperity. It's beneficial to shift our focus away from comparisons and instead direct our energy toward praising and serving God, utilizing the unique gifts we have been given. This approach can lead to a more fulfilling and joyful life, rooted in faith and gratitude.

Comparing danger

Comparing ourselves to others can indeed be a risky endeavor. It often leads to feelings of inadequacy, jealousy, or dissatisfaction. Each person's journey is unique, shaped by their circumstances, experiences, and choices. When we focus on comparisons, we may overlook our own strengths and the progress we've made.

It's essential to recognize that everyone faces their own struggles, even if they aren't visible on the surface. Instead of comparing, fostering a mindset of self-acceptance and gratitude for our individual paths can be more beneficial. This approach encourages personal growth and helps us appreciate the unique qualities and gifts we each possess. Ultimately, focusing on our own journey allows us to live more fulfilling lives.

Chapter Twelve

When We Praise ...

At times, we may struggle to praise the Lord, especially when faced with numerous trials. The adversary often distracts us, prompting complaints instead of worship. We may find ourselves fixated on what remains unfulfilled rather than reflecting on the blessings we've received. Yet, the Word reminds us, "When you pass through the waters, I will be with you; and when you pass through the rivers, they will not sweep over you. When you walk through the fire, you will not be burned; the flames will not set you ablaze" (Isaiah 43:2).

Praising God can lead to our liberation. Take, for example, the apostle Paul. While imprisoned, he chose to worship the Lord rather than succumb to despair. In an environment far from conducive to praise, he lifted his voice in worship, trusting in God's presence. His act of worship led to miraculous freedom as the prison doors swung open.

I find great joy in worshipping the Lord. Throughout the many dark times I've faced, worship brings illumination to my spirit. Even when circumstances seem bleak, an inner peace envelops me when I praise Him. It's remarkable how, in the midst of struggle, we can find comfort and serenity through worship.

I find myself worshiping Him in spirit, even when circumstances do not seemingly change. The presence of the Lord in my life brings me such joy that I become oblivious to everything but Him. I often wish I could dedicate the entire night to worship. On my days off, I sometimes spend one or two hours kneeling in prayer.

I express my worship through hymns, singing praises such as:

• "Who Has No Equal Nor Rival"
• "Lives Enthroned on a Throne Eternal"
• "In the Midst of His Assembly I Sing His Praise"
• "Even in the Midst of a Multitude of People, Saying, You Are Great, You Are Great."

When I listen to Lili's spiritual songs, I join in worship with her, praising God together. I have learned that every mountain will be brought low through worship and praise, allowing me to see only what is heavenly. In those moments, I immediately enter into the Lord's presence.

I recall a time during my chemotherapy treatment when I felt the Lord's presence deeply. I began to weep and pray in tongues. A nurse quickly approached me and gently wiped my tears with a cotton pad, cautioning, "You should not weep; if you do so within 48 hours after a chemo treatment, it could cause your skin to peel." Yet, feeling the touch of the Spirit of God, I continued to worship, tears streaming down my face onto my chest. I thought to myself that if my face was going to suffer while worshiping my beloved God, then so be it.

It is important to recognize that adversities may arise to deter us from worshiping God. The enemy does not want us to worship because he fears its power and influence. We should remember that true worship can lead to transformation, just as Jonah was released from the fish's belly immediately after he turned to God in praise.

I find myself worshiping Him in Spirit, even when circumstances do not change. The presence of the Lord in my life fills me with such joy that I become oblivious to everything but Him. Sometimes, I wish I could worship through the night. On my days off, I often spend one to two hours kneeling in prayer.

I sing hymns of praise to the Lord, including:

• "Who Has No Equal Nor Rival"
• "Lives Enthroned on a Throne Eternal"

131

- "In the Midst of His Assembly I Sing His Praise"
- "Even in the Midst of a Multitude of People, Saying, You Are Great, You Are Great."

When I play Lili's spiritual songs, I immediately join her in worship and praise God together. I have learned that every mountain will be brought low through worship and praise, allowing me to see only what is heavenly. In those moments, I enter the Lord's presence right away.

I remember a time during my chemotherapy treatments when I felt the Lord's presence strongly. I began to weep and pray in tongues, and a nurse quickly approached me, wiping my tears with a cotton pad. She cautioned, "You should not weep; if you do so within 48 hours after a chemotherapy treatment, it could cause your skin to peel." However, feeling the touch of the Spirit of God, I continued to worship, tears streaming down my face and dripping onto my chest. I thought that if my face was going to suffer while worshiping my beloved God, so be it.

It is crucial to recognize that the enemy may bring obstacles to deter us from worshiping God. He fears the power of worship because he does not want us to praise God. We should remember that true worship can lead to transformation; just as Jonah was released from the fish's belly immediately after he turned to God in praise.

Jonah said, "But I, with shouts of grateful praise, will sacrifice to you. What I have vowed I will do good. I will say, 'Salvation comes from the Lord.'" (Jonah 2:9-10). Regardless of the challenges we face, we should strive to praise God, even when certain circumstances may hinder us. In worship, we can find answers, experience release, and see doors that have remained closed begin to open. Worship and praise have the power to help us overcome.

At times, our suffering may intensify as we praise and worship the Lord. I recall my mother, who experienced significant hardships throughout her life yet remained devoted to the Lord. Despite facing many trials that could have led her to complain, she consistently chose to praise and worship Him. The greater her suffering, the more she sought comfort in fasting, prayer, and praise. There was a period when my father endured severe pain due to multiple illnesses, and she took on the responsibility of caring for him. While there were other challenges she faced that I hesitate to share, her unwavering commitment to praising the Lord was evident.

At times, we experience suffering because the Lord has a purpose for us. This purpose may involve becoming examples for others or offering help in their times of need. In the midst of our struggles, it can be difficult to see the bigger picture that God has for us. However, once we move past the hardships, we may come to understand that our experiences were intended to lead us to a particular realization or outcome. Reflecting on my own journey, I realize I might not have had the motivation to write this book had I not faced my own challenges.

I often found myself thinking, "My suffering is nothing compared to what others are enduring," especially when I observed people facing severe difficulties such as financial problems,family issues, marital issues, mental health challenges while I was contending with cancer and various afflictions.

Instead of succumbing to worry, we should place our trust in God and turn to worship during such challenging times. This aligns with the message in Philippians 4:6-7: "The Lord is near. Do not be anxious about anything, but in every situation, by prayer and petition, with thanksgiving, present your requests to God. And the peace of God, which transcends all understanding, will guard your hearts and your minds in Christ Jesus." Our Father is always near, and it is not with bitterness, but with gratitude, that we should offer our prayers and supplications to God.

When we focus on praising the Lord, our attention shifts away from ourselves and our suffering. With our hope anchored in Him, it is appropriate for our eyes to be fixed on God. He deserves our praise, regardless of our daily experiences. As stated in Psalm 150:2, "Praise him for his mighty acts; praise him according to his excellent greatness."

Praising the Lord guides us toward a life of humility, reminding us that He is our support as the Creator and King of the world.

Additionally, the act of praise can have significant spiritual effects, as it is believed that adversarial forces will retreat in response to worshiping God. The story of Jehoshaphat demonstrates this power; God miraculously defeated the enemies of Judah when they chose to praise Him. As they sang and worshiped, God intervened by setting ambushes against the Ammonites, Moabites, and the inhabitants of Mount Seir, leading to their defeat.

In 2 Chronicles 20:20-22, Jehoshaphat encouraged the people, saying, "Believe in the Lord your God, and you shall be established; believe His prophets, and you shall prosper." He appointed singers to lead in worship, proclaiming, "Praise the Lord, for His mercy endures forever." Their collective act of singing and praising prompted a decisive action from God against their adversaries.

These examples illustrate that praise is not only an expression of gratitude but also a means to invite God's presence and power into our circumstances.

When the people of Judah began to praise God, their enemies were defeated, and they were able to seize the spoils. This illustrates that we should praise the Lord regardless of our circumstances, as praise can lead to significant blessings and victories.

My Prayer

"My Lord, I ask for your help for those who are enduring various afflictions and find it difficult to praise you in those moments. Thank you for your faithfulness, protection, perfect love, and power. We depend on you regardless of our circumstances and appreciate all your goodness and kindness. When challenges arise and darkness surrounds us, remind us of your word. Grant us the strength to keep our eyes fixed on you at all times. We are grateful for your presence and for providing us with everything we need. In Jesus Christ's name, I pray; Amen."

REMEMBER Praising God offers numerous benefits that can positively impact both individuals and communities.

1. Spiritual Connection: Praise fosters a deeper relationship with God, helping individuals feel more connected to their faith and spiritual beliefs.

2. Emotional Uplift: Engaging in praise can lead to feelings of joy, gratitude, and peace, helping to alleviate stress and anxiety.

3. Perspective Shift: Praising God can shift focus away from personal challenges, encouraging a more positive outlook and greater resilience in difficult situations.

4. Community and Unity: Congregational praise can strengthen bonds within a community, fostering a sense of belonging and support among believers.

5. Encouragement and Motivation: Acts of praise can inspire others, providing encouragement and motivation in their own spiritual journeys.

6. Gratitude and Reflection: Regularly expressing praise encourages individuals to reflect on their blessings and cultivate an attitude of gratitude.

Overall, praising God can enhance spiritual well-being and promote a fulfilling and positive life experience.

Chapter Thirteen

Mental Disease and Depression

One day, while I was in a mall trying on clothes to buy, a lady stared at me; I felt scared because I had never experienced someone looking at me like that before.

When I entered a fitting room to try on the clothes, she followed me inside.

I grcctcd hcr, my apprehension evident. "Are you Habesha?" she asked.

"Yes, I am. Is there anything I can help you with?" I responded.

She replied, "Yes, you can help me with many things."

"Let's start with the small things for now," I suggested, continuing, "But you have to wait for me until I finish trying on the clothes."

"If you're willing, I can go in with you and help you with the trial," she offered.
"Okay," I agreed.

As I tried on the clothes, I asked her, "Why were you staring at me?"

She looked down and said, "I heard a voice saying, 'Talk to that lady,' and I was following you, but you didn't see me." "Okay, what is it that you want me to help you with?" I inquired.

Unable to hold back her tears, she began to cry. As her tears flowed, she transformed before my eyes. I wiped her tears with my coat since I didn't have a handkerchief and said, "Let's get out of here. I can buy the clothes some other day." We left the fitting room and began to walk slowly.

"I have a mental illness," she confided. "It's been a long time since I became sick, but no one has been able to understand me. My husband says to me, 'Are you going insane again?' Strangely, he is a Protestant. I used to go to church, but one day I fell ill and was prayed for at a church conference. Then everyone started talking about me, saying they had long suspected that I was demon-possessed. I gave up attending church because I was deeply hurt."

There was a woman who suffered from mental illness, similar to my own experiences. When I confided in her about my struggles, she cautioned me not to share my challenges with anyone, especially Christians. She explained that some believe a Christian cannot experience mental illness unless they are demon-possessed. As a result, they may not view individuals with mental health issues as whole persons and may label them as "insane." After sharing my story, I found myself isolated, as I struggled to find anyone who could help me. She advised me to be careful about who I confide in, to prevent experiencing what had happened to her.

This woman also spoke about a man she knew who dealt with depression. She mentioned that he sometimes used smoking and drinking as a way to dull his senses. She expressed the desire for someone who would accept her and offer kindness instead of judgment, saying what she truly needed was compassion, not a reminder that her depression was a sign of demon possession.

I thanked her for sharing her story and told her that I loved her. I offered my phone number, suggesting she could find support in our church, where many people face similar challenges. I could accompany her to seek help or even take her home. However, she requested that I keep her situation confidential, indicating she didn't want others to know about her struggles. I agreed, and we parted ways.

Ultimately, this woman overcome her depression and is now serving the Lord.

There was a woman named Fernanda whom I knew many years ago while working at an organization called Young Missionary. The employees there were believers, and Fernanda had dedicated her life to missionary work. Her husband was also a notable figure in the ministry. At that time, I was a young girl, and Fernanda, being older, often provided me with advice and prayers.

Fernanda had five children and came from Brazil, where both she and her husband had a significant impact through their work. When you entered their home, the presence of God was often felt, and her prayers always brought me a sense of happiness. Her husband served as a pastor, and her father-in-law was a well-respected pastor in Brazil.

One day, Fernanda showed me a video of her father-in-law preaching. As I watched, I became engrossed by the way the Lord worked through him and remarked, "I will see this great minister of the Lord someday." Fernanda replied, "He has passed away." I was taken aback and asked, "What happened to him?" She responded, "He committed suicide."

Given that he was a Christian who had been used mightily by the Lord, I found it difficult to comprehend. I asked Fernanda if she was sure, and she confirmed, "Yes, I am." She then explained that he had experienced serious mental illness that went unrecognized by those around him, including his wife. After years of ministry, he faced significant spiritual battles, but when he shared his struggles, people often dismissed his experiences, insisting, "Satan is fighting you; you cannot be mentally ill because you are a Christian."

Some church elders excommunicated him for six months, believing, "How can he pray for us when he is unable to save himself? He might even transfer his spirit of depression to us. He should be excommunicated to prevent his spirit of depression from affecting us." Despite this, he continued to travel through villages, preaching the gospel.

Fernanda expressed her confusion, stating, "I do not understand why we, as Christians, prevent people from seeking help by associating mental illness with Satan. My husband and I are currently engaged in providing assistance to those dealing with such issues." At the time, I didn't fully grasp the challenges of mental illness. However, over time,

I came to understand the importance of addressing it, especially after witnessing many individuals receiving help. Sadly, I also heard stories like, "They committed suicide," and found that many of these individuals were church-goers. It was particularly alarming to learn about young people who had taken their own lives.

As I write this book, I can't help but wonder how many ministers of God may have succumbed to depression without anyone reaching out to help them. A close relative of mine experienced depression, and unfortunately, no one was able to assist him. Despite his deep faith in the Lord, he passed away due to a lack of support, as both ministers and laypeople often struggle to understand the complexities of this disease.

Recently, a young preacher named Astar Andrew Stoecklein took his own life, leaving behind his three children and wife, after preaching about depression. A well-known pastor from a mega church, Pastor Jim Howard, also ended his life. These tragic events underscore that mental illness can affect anyone. While other illnesses are often treated promptly, mental illness is frequently misunderstood and stigmatized. In many Christian communities, conditions like depression are sometimes perceived as attacks from Satan. Some ministers believe that genuine Christians cannot experience mental illness, thinking that such conditions indicate a lack of faith or possession by evil.

This is a critical issue that requires serious attention within our broader community and especially in the church. It is essential that we pray for those who are struggling with mental health issues and offer them as much support as possible. Encouragement and compassion are vital in these situations.

I recall a young woman who lived in America. After accepting Jesus Christ as her personal savior, she faced a severe battle with depression. One night, she reached out to me, expressing her despair and stating that she was considering suicide. I asked her why she wasn't receiving support as a worship leader. She responded that many people were unaware of the realities of depression and had dismissed her struggles, labeling her as demon-possessed instead.

This illustrates a significant gap in understanding mental health within some communities. Rather than offering support and understanding, individuals suffering from depression often face judgment. It is crucial that we approach such individuals with love and compassion, recognizing the need for genuine assistance and care, rather than labeling them as simply "mentally ill."

The issue of suicide among youth, particularly those aged 15 to 20, is a serious concern stemming from depression. A particularly memorable and tragic case from our community involved a 19-year-old who ended his life by dousing himself in kerosene and setting himself on fire.

This deeply saddened me and raised the question, "How distressed must he have been to make such a decision?"

Often, when young people express feelings of depression to their parents, they may not receive the help they need. Instead, parents may respond with frustration or misunderstanding, asking, "Why are you depressed? What do you lack?" Such responses can make their children reluctant to open up, leading them to suffer in silence.

It is essential to approach individuals experiencing depression with compassion and understanding, ensuring they do not feel stigmatized. Both the church as an organization and individuals within the community have a responsibility to support those who are struggling. Offering love, understanding, and earnest prayer, rather than judgment, can make a significant difference.

As the apostle Paul expressed in his letters, "We are hard-pressed on every side, yet not crushed; we are perplexed, but not in despair; persecuted, but not forsaken; struck down, but not destroyed" (2 Corinthians 4:8-10). This emphasizes resilience in the face of adversity.

It is important to recognize that feelings of isolation and unworthiness can be exacerbated by negative influences. By cultivating a supportive environment, we can help individuals feel protected and loved, reducing the stigma surrounding mental health and encouraging open dialogue.

Many individuals may feel unqualified or unloved at times, leading to feelings of despair and darkness. This despair can contribute to depression. It's important to recognize that negative thoughts can stem from adversarial influences.

According to Romans 8:37, "In all these things we are more than conquerors through him who loved us." Additionally, Jesus states in John 10:10, "The thief comes only to steal and kill and destroy; I have come that they may have life, and have it to the full." This indicates that while negative forces may seek to harm us, there is also a promise of life and fulfillment.

Understanding the tactics of adverse influences can help us remain vigilant. It is widely acknowledged that many negative experiences and struggles are attributed to these forces. Depression may indeed be viewed as both a spiritual challenge and a mental health issue. Keeping this perspective in mind, it is essential to provide support to those who are facing these struggles.

A review of biblical accounts shows that many of God's people faced significant trials. For instance, David, who is described as "a man after my heart," shared his struggles with God, saying, "Record my misery; put my tears in your wineskin; are they not in your record?" (Psalm 56:8). Similarly, Moses, feeling the weight of his responsibilities toward the people of Israel, implored God, "Please go ahead and kill me if I have found favor in your eyes, and do not let me face my own ruin" (Numbers 11:15). These examples reflect the profound challenges faced by individuals in their journeys.

By acknowledging these struggles and offering compassion and support, we can help others navigate their own challenges effectively.

The Biblical accounts of Elijah and Moses illustrate that even the most faithful individuals can experience deep despair and contemplate ending their lives. In 1 Kings 19:3-4, we read about Elijah's fear and his plea to God, stating, "I have had enough, LORD. Take my life; I am no better than my ancestors." This reveals the profound weight of his struggles, showcasing that feelings of hopelessness can affect anyone, regardless of their spiritual standing.

These accounts remind us that the experiences of suffering and sadness are part of the human condition. The Bible does not shy away from presenting these moments of vulnerability, nor does it convey judgment for them. Rather, it highlights the importance of compassion and understanding towards those who are struggling.

Sadly, stigma often surrounds mental health issues, leading to misconceptions that can alienate those who need help the most. Instead of offering support, some may mistakenly label individuals facing mental health challenges as flawed or unworthy, saying things like "He is not a Christian; he is from Satan." This perspective can prevent individuals from seeking the help they need and can increase feelings of isolation.

It is essential to approach those experiencing depression and mental health challenges with empathy and an open heart. By fostering a supportive environment, we can encourage individuals to share their struggles without fear of judgment. This approach not only helps in addressing their needs but also contributes to reducing the stigma surrounding mental health. Offering kindness, understanding, and resources can make a significant difference in the lives of those who are suffering.

In reflecting on these issues, we are reminded of our responsibility to support one another and to approach those in distress with compassion and a willingness to listen.

is true that mental health challenges, particularly depress-ion, can significantly impact not only the individu-als who experience them but also their families and close relationships. Often, those struggling with depression may find it difficult to acknowledge their condition, leading to feelings of isolation and reluctance to seek help. This reluctance can create strain within families, as loved ones might feel overwhelmed or helpless in supporting someone who is unwilling to admit their struggles.

In such situations, it is important for family members to approach their loved ones with compassion and understand-ing. Encouraging open and non-judgmental communication can help create a safe space for the individual to share their feelings. It can be beneficial for spouses to collaborate in seeking help, whether through prayer, supportive dialogue, or professional intervention. This combined effort can be vital in navigating the complexities of mental health issues.

The example of a seemingly perfect couple, who appear to have no problems, serves as a reminder that mental health struggles can be hidden beneath the surface, regardless of outward appearances. It highlights the importance of recognizing that everyone has their own battles, and those who seem fine may be experiencing profound challenges.

In summary, fostering a supportive environment and encouraging individuals to seek help can make a positive difference. Communities, including faith-based groups, play a crucial role in promoting understanding and providing resources for those facing mental health issues, ultimately contributing to a healthier support system for both individuals and their families.

In our community, the individuals who bear the greatest burden related to depression are often the closest family members of those affected. Many individuals struggling with depression are reluctant to acknowledge their condition, which can place a significant strain on their relatives. I have witnessed this firsthand. They may fear that admitting they have depression will lead to judgment from others, causing them to withdraw further. This reluctance can create considerable challenges for spouses and children.

As members of the Christian community, we should strive to support those grappling with depression to the best of our ability until they find a solution.

Spouses should avoid sharing their partner's struggles with anyone else. Instead, they can focus on providing support through prayer and, when necessary, encouraging their loved one to seek professional help from a psychiatrist.

For example, I once knew a devoted Christian couple who regularly attended church. They had beautiful children and were both highly educated. From the outside, they seemed to have no problems at all.

During one of our prayer sessions at church, the wife of an evangelist unexpectedly began convulsing and screaming, which startled a sister and me. Her husband, visibly distressed, turned to the pastor and said tearfully, "I think it is getting worse now." The pastor responded with assurance, "Be strong. The demon living in her will leave, and you will find peace." At that time, I struggled to comprehend many things happening around me. Although I felt the need to remain silent due to my confusion, I also found myself asking questions.

I had a deep affection for this woman, so I approached her husband to ask, "What has happened to her?" He replied, "You are just a child; this is beyond your understanding." I defended myself by saying, "I am 20 years old. Why do you consider me a child?" Most members of the church I attended were middle-aged, and they often viewed me as younger and less experienced. Despite this, my curiosity led me to tell him, "I want to talk with you." He responded, "She will talk to you herself."

The following week, I waited for her and said, "I want to talk with you today." She replied, "Wongeliye, I am too sick to talk today. If you would like, you can come to my home another day."

After the church program, I sought out her husband and inquired, "What has happened to your wife?" He responded by saying, "My wife has severe depression; no one else knows except our pastor. She frightens me when she says, 'I will commit suicide.' I often ask her, 'Who will take care of me and the children if you go?' That usually calms her, but now her condition has worsened. She isn't working anymore, and I am afraid to leave her alone."

Curious, I asked, "What is the solution then?" He replied, "It is prayer. She needs companionship; she wants someone to talk to and someone who can uplift her." I suggested, "Why don't I come to your home? I can talk to her." He agreed and asked me to call her.

I shared this with another sister, saying, "Let us go together." She responded, "Going there uninvited—isn't that a bit awkward? What will we say if asked why we're there?" I reassured her, "Don't worry. I will handle the conversation tonight." She added, "By the way, the woman loves you; she may be more willing to talk with you."

The next day, we visited her home. We were warmly welcomed and sat down to talk. She began sharing about her children, and while she spoke highly of her husband, she felt it wasn't enough. She described how attentive, comforting, and understanding he was, emphasizing that he never judged her. My companion and I expressed our admiration for him and his support.

At one point, my friend asked her, "What does it feel like? What are the symptoms of your illness?" She replied, "What I'm about to tell you may be hard to understand; it's something that not many can grasp. I have this overwhelming impulse to scream and to commit suicide. Despite being well-educated and hearing from my husband that I'm attractive, there's a persistent voice that torments me, telling me I'm empty and that ending my life would be preferable." She mentioned that her husband had taken her to the hospital twice, where healthcare professionals informed him that she had a severe mental illness, warning him that it would be challenging for both him and their children. They advised that she needed serious follow-up care and suggested that she should be admitted to a psychiatric hospital. We acknowledged this recommendation but did not proceed with it.

She continued, expressing a reluctance to go to any hospital and stating, "The only solution I see is prayer, but I don't want to pray right now. My husband prays for me." Then she asked us to wait and left the room, not returning immediately as she had fallen asleep.

After arriving home from work, the husband checked on her and informed us, "She is sleeping in our late son's room; he might have been on her mind while she was talking with you." I was surprised and asked, "Did you have a son who has now passed away?" He replied, "Yes, and it's partly because of him that she suffers from depression. She believes she is to blame; our son had been asleep for several hours, and she thought to herself, 'He must be really tired today,' and let him sleep without waking him. Later, she wondered why he was sleeping for so long and went to check on him, only to find that he had passed away. Since then, she has struggled with guilt and depression. When her depression worsens, she often enters his room, screams, and weeps, not wanting to leave. Please pray for her that she wakes up feeling better."

It's important to recognize that mental illness requires a combination of prayer, professional help, ongoing support, and love. Individuals experiencing mental health challenges need compassionate people who love and support them, without judgment, and who can understand their feelings.

Many Christians may not realize that they can also experience depression. This misconception can lead individuals to feel ashamed or fearful about seeking help, causing them to isolate themselves. Once isolated, they may become more vulnerable to negative thoughts and feelings, including despair and hopelessness. It's crucial to address these issues with empathy and understanding.

I have explained what depression is; but hereafter we will look at what is expected of us and what people with depression should do to come out of it.

Helping individuals who are experiencing depression, as well as empowering them to help themselves, can involve several steps: How We Can Help Depressed Individuals:

1. Listen Actively:- Offer non-judgmental ears and let them express their feelings. Sometimes, just being heard can provide comfort.

2. Encourage Professional Help: —Suggest seeking support from a mental health professional, such as a therapist or counselor, who can provide appropriate treatment and guidance.

3. Be Supportive: Offer your support by checking in regularly and being available to help with daily tasks when needed.

4. Educate Yourself: Learn about depression to better understand what they are going through and how best to support them

5. Promote Healthy Habits: Encourage a balanced lifestyle, including regular exercise, a nutritious diet, and sufficient sleep, as these can positively impact mental health.

6. Avoid Judgment: Be patient and avoid making judgments about their feelings or behaviors.

Though praying for the victims of depression is necessary, the problem cannot be solved through prayer alone; there are somethings which we need to do. Among them are:

Understanding and empathy can go a long way. How Individuals Can Help Themselves:

1. Seek Professional Help: Consulting a mental health professional can provide the necessary tools and strategies for managing depression.

2. Practice Self-Care: –Engage in self-care activities that promote relaxation and well-being, such as mindfulness, meditation, or hobbies.

3. Establish a Routine: Creating a daily schedule can provide structure and a sense of accomplishment.

4. Connect with Others: Reach out to friends, family, or support groups. Social connections can provide a sense of belonging and support.

5. Set Small Goals: Break tasks into manageable steps and set achievable goals to foster a sense of progress and motivation.

6. Challenge Negative Thoughts: Work on recognizing and reframing negative thought patterns through cognitive behavioral techniques.

7. Stay Active: Incorporate physical activity into daily life, as exercise can help improve mood and reduce symptoms of depression.

8. Limit Substance Use: Reduce or eliminate the use of alcohol and drugs, as these can exacerbate depressive symptoms.

How can the mentally ill help themselves:

1. Professional Help: Engaging with mental health professionals, such as psychologists, psychiatrists, or counselors, can provide individuals with tailored support, therapy, and medication if necessary.

2. Peer Support: —-Connecting with others who have similar experiences can create a sense of community and understanding. Support groups, both in-person and online, allow individuals to share their feelings and coping strategies.

3. Self-Help Strategies: Individuals can explore various self-help techniques, such as mindfulness, meditation, journaling, or engaging in hobbies, to manage their mental health.

4. Education and Awareness: Increasing knowledge about mental health can reduce stigma and empower individuals to seek help. This includes understanding symptoms, treatment options, and resources available.

5. Crisis Resources: In times of urgent need, crisis hotlines and emergency services can provide immediate support and intervention for those in distress.

6. Lifestyle Adjustments: Encouraging healthy lifestyle choices, such as proper nutrition, regular physical activity, and sufficient sleep, can positively impact mental well-being.

How can we help someone with mental illness?

Helping someone who is experiencing mental health challenges requires Sensitivity, understanding, and practical support. Here are some neutral steps to consider:

1. Educate Yourself ***Learn about mental health issues to better understand what the person is experiencing. Familiarize yourself with symptoms, treatments, and common misconceptions.

2. Listen Actively ***Offer a listening ear without judgment. Let them express their feelings and thoughts openly, and validate their experiences.

3. Encourage Professional Help ***Suggest seeking assistance from a mental health professional, such as a therapist or counselor, if they are open to it.

4. Be Supportive ***Offer your support and let them know you are there for them. This can include checking in regularly or offering to accompany them to appointments.

5. Promote Self-Care *** Encourage activities that promote well-being, such as exercise, healthy eating, and getting enough sleep. Suggest engaging in hobbies or activities they enjoy.

6. Respect Their Space *** Understand that they may need time alone. Respect their boundaries while making it clear that you are available if they want to talk or need support.

7. Avoid Judgment *** Be non-judgmental in your responses. Avoid making assumptions about their feelings or experiences, and refrain from giving unsolicited advice.

8. Encourage Healthy Routines • Help them establish a daily routine that includes structure and balance, as this can contribute to stability and a sense of control.

9. Watch for Warning Signs • Be aware of potential signs of worsening mental health, such as changes in behavior, mood, or withdrawal from activities. If you notice concerning changes, consider discussing them with the person.

10. Be Patient *** Recovery and coping can take time. Be patient and understanding, recognizing that progress may be gradual and nonlinear.

11. Respect Confidentiality * **Maintain trust by keeping conversations confidential unless there is a risk of harm to themselves or others.

12. Encourage Social Connections *** Help them maintain connections with friends and family. Social support can be crucial for their well-being. By providing support in these ways, you can help create a positive environment for someone dealing with mental health challenges. Remember that each individual is different, so tailoring your approach based on their specific needs and preferences is essential.[1]

Postpartum Depression (PPD)

Postpartum depression is a type of depression that can occur after childbirth. Many women may experience changes in their mood, emotions, and physical well-being during this time. For some, these changes can signal the onset of postpartum depression.

I have personally experienced this issue. I found myself crying frequently, feeling easily irritated, and becoming annoyed by minor issues.

---

[1] Regarding depression and mental health, I accessed mental health resources, including AHS Adult Services. The CMHA Calgary builds awareness of Mental Health (healing with compassion) and I also conducted my own online research.

At first, I did not realize that I had postpartum depression. As my symptoms worsened, I decided to visit my doctor. During the consultation, he asked, "What seems to be the problem?" I responded, "I feel irritated by every little thing; I struggle with the desire to change or engage with others; I often feel anger without a clear reason; and I cry for no apparent reason." He informed me that I was experiencing postpartum depression and prescribed medication. However, I was hesitant to take the medication.

Later that day, I was watching the news when I heard a report about a well-known doctor who took her own life by jumping in front of a moving train while carrying her son in Toronto. The report revealed that she had been suffering from postpartum depression, but no one was aware of her struggles. Upon hearing this news, I felt terrified and began to waver between the decision to take the medication prescribed by my doctor or to avoid it. I turned to prayer, asking God for help: "Oh, Lord, I do not want to take this medicine; please guide me."

Prior to this incident, I had nurses visiting to check on me. I asked them if I should take the medication, and they advised me to do so, warning that avoiding it could lead to a dangerous condition. They mentioned that even well-known individuals can fall victim to this type of depression.

I do not want anyone experiencing depression to struggle in silence, which is why I choose to share my past challenges openly. Some may argue that those who suffer from depression are not true Christians, and I have encountered similar sentiments. When I expressed my feelings to those who came to support me, they often said, "You are a Christian; rebuke it in the name of Jesus. Postpartum depression is merely a manifestation of evil; do not accept it."

I realized that it was difficult for some people to grasp what I was experiencing, as they often equated all struggles to spiritual warfare. This perspective can be hurtful for individuals facing depression. I chose to leave my struggles in the hands of the Lord, understanding that not everyone can comprehend the depths of someone's pain, regardless of their beliefs.

One day, we visited a sister who had recently given birth. When we arrived, we noticed her house was messy. Even though she knew we were coming, she hadn't tidied up. There were two other guests already there, but they seemed to be sitting idly. The sister who accompanied me was close to the new mother, so she started cleaning up the house. After tidying up, she asked her, "Your hair is uncombed, your house is messy, and you have bloodshot eyes. Are you alright?"

The new mother replied, "I don't know what has happened to me; I feel easily annoyed, I yell at my husband, I don't want to nurse my baby, I'm experiencing a loss of appetite, I cannot concentrate, and I feel confused." I responded, "You might be experiencing a form of depression known as postpartum depression, which can occur after childbirth, but it is treatable."

As soon as I said this, the two other women reacted with frustration and said, "What kind of depression are you talking about? We are Christians; such things cannot affect us." I asked, "Then why is she showing these symptoms?" They responded, "It's a battle with Satan; he never stops trying to fight us."

I said to them, "Whether we call it a fight or depression, one thing is certain: this woman needs healing, and she can receive that healing only when we accept the reality of the issue and pray about it." They replied, "Why are you so quick to advise her to seek treatment? Are you a doctor?" I explained that I had experienced it myself and that I faced many challenges as a result of not seeking help immediately. This prompted a silence among them.

After a brief moment, the new mother asked me, "How did you cope with the depression that can occur after childbirth, known as postpartum depression?" I shared my experiences with her, and she found comfort in my story. After we prayed together, we took our leave. As David said in Psalm 94:10, "When anxiety was great within me, your consolation brought me joy." God's comfort truly brings peace and joy to the heart.

I want to emphasize that postpartum depression (PPD) should not be taken lightly. Many mothers experience this condition shortly after childbirth. Often, it is associated with Satan, and within our community, it is frequently dismissed. There is particularly a lack of understanding about PPD among believers. I would like to outline below some solutions to help identify and assist mothers struggling with this condition. It's important to note that this issue cannot be resolved solely through fasting and prayer. With that in mind, let's explore what steps we can take based on research and insights from experts in the field.

Here are some solutions for addressing postpartum depression (PPD):

1. Education and Awareness: Understand the signs and symptoms of postpartum depression. Being informed can help in recognizing early warning signals.

2. Prenatal Care: Attend regular prenatal check-ups and discuss any mental health history with your healthcare provider to create a tailored support plan.

3. Build a Support Network: Establish a strong support system that includes family, friends, or support groups. Having people to talk to and share experiences with can be beneficial.

4. Communicate Openly: Encourage open communication with your partner, family, and friends about your feelings and experiences. Expressing emotions can help alleviate stress.

5. Practice Self-Care: Prioritize self-care by ensuring adequate rest, nutrition, and physical activity. Engaging in activities that bring you joy can also be helpful.

6. Set Realistic Expectations: Acknowledge that adjusting to motherhood can be challenging. Setting realistic expectations about parenting and seeking help when needed can help reduce pressure.

7. Seek Professional Help: If feelings of sadness, anxiety, or overwhelm persist, do not hesitate to reach out to a mental health professional. Early intervention can make a significant difference.

8. Limit Stressors: Identify and reduce sources of stress where possible. This may include delegating tasks or declining additional responsibilities during the postpartum period.

9. Stay Connected: Maintain social connections, even if it's through phone calls or online interactions. Isolation can worsen feelings of depression.

10. Mindfulness and Relaxation Techniques • Practice mindfulness, meditation, or relaxation techniques to manage stress and promote emotional well-being.

11. Join Support Groups • Consider joining a postpartum support group where you can connect with others experiencing similar challenges. Sharing experiences can be comforting.

12. Monitor Mental Health • Keep track of mental and emotional well-being. If there are any concerning changes, address them promptly with a healthcare provider. By taking these steps, new mothers can foster a supportive environment that may help prevent or mitigate the effects of postpartum depression. It's essential to prioritize mental health and seek help when needed.

How Can We Help Individuals Who Have Postpartum depression?

Postpartum support is essential for new mothers as they transition into parenthood.

1. Emotional Support • Providing a listening ear and understanding from family, friends, and support groups can help mothers feel less isolated.

2. Professional Help • Access to mental health professionals, such as therapists or counselors, who specialize in postpartum issues, can be beneficial for managing any emotional challenges.

3. Education and Resources • Offering information about postpartum depression and other related conditions can empower mothers to recognize symptoms and seek help early.

4. Physical Support • Assistance with daily tasks, such as cooking, cleaning, or childcare, can alleviate stress and allow mothers to focus on recovery and bonding with their baby.

5. Support Groups • Participating in support groups for new mothers can provide a sense of community and   shared

experiences, helping to normalize the challenges of motherhood.

6. Encouragement of Self-Care • Encouraging mothers to prioritize self-care, including rest, nutrition, and personal time, is vital for overall well-being.

7. Communication • Open lines of communication with partners and loved ones about feelings, challenges, and needs can foster a supportive environment.

8. Regular Check-ins • Regular check-ins from family or friends can help monitor the mother's emotional health and provide an opportunity for her to express any concerns.
9. Access to Resources • Providing information about local resources, such as parenting classes, lactation consultants, or mental health services, can help mothers navigate their postpartum journey.

10. Understanding and Patience • Offering understanding and patience as new mothers adjust to their roles can alleviate feelings of inadequacy or overwhelm. By focusing on these areas, postpartum support can significantly

contribute to the well-being of new mothers and help them navigate the challenges of this transitional period.[2]

---

[2] Regarding the postponement of depression treatment: Information provided by my nurse and doctor . Based on that information, I have included this note, and also conducted my own online research. TV shows , articles such as feelings of sadness anxiety unrealistic expectations such as the year 2000-2005.

Chapter Fourteen

Fear

In our modern age, many individuals experience worry and fear about various aspects of life. The phrase "Do not fear" appears in the Bible over 300 times, yet feelings of anxiety persist. Personally, I have faced significant fears, particularly related to exams and class presentations. Public speaking was another source of considerable anxiety for me. When asked to provide testimony or talk about specific topics, including the children I teach, I would often feel overwhelmed to the point of being unable to speak. During interviews, I sometimes forgot what I knew, yet I was fortunate to receive encouragement from my interviewers, which helped me through those experiences.

Fear affects each of us in different ways. Many people worry about financial issues or the possibility of losing their jobs. Some may feel anxious about forming close relationships, while others fear pregnancy or the health of their future children. Concerns can also arise regarding children's behavior, leading to questions such as, "What if they don't grow up to be responsible adults?" or "What if they engage in risky behaviors?"

Health concerns can trigger anxiety as well; for example, being asked by a doctor for an examination can provoke fear. Specific phobias, such as a fear of dogs or flying, are common, as is anxiety about the future, with questions like, "What will happen to me tomorrow?" Ultimately, many individuals grapple with fear stemming from these concerns or other personal experiences.

Particularly in the present time, many individuals struggle with fears that can make even simple tasks, like going outside, feel daunting. When fear strikes, it becomes crucial to turn to the Lord and pray, invoking Scripture rather than succumbing to idle worry.

I recall a story from a sister who shared her concerns about her husband. He harbored an intense fear of nearly everything, including their neighbors, despite lacking any logical reasons for such apprehensions. She recounted, "He would spend nights peering out the window, convinced that our new neighbors had a menacing demeanor and didn't like people of color." Even the slightest sound would trigger his anxiety, prompting him to exclaim in panic, "A thief has broken into our house!"

She noted that when it snowed, neither of them would drive, as he feared the roads. Additionally, she felt compelled to keep the curtains drawn, fearing that even this small act

174

might invite scrutiny from outsiders. She expressed her growing concern that his fears were beginning to affect her as well.

In response, I asked her, "How can he be so fearful while serving the Lord?" She replied, "It seems that it is God's servants that Satan seeks to attack. How can you, a minister of the Gospel, question his fears?" I acknowledged her perspective and stated, "It seems your husband's feelings might be rooted not just in fear but also in anxiety. While it is natural to be afraid of specific things, it's concerning when one is afraid of so many different aspects of life."

It is clearly stated in the Bible that people of God, including figures like David, have faced fear. However, it is important to recognize that fear can sometimes develop into more severe forms of anxiety.

The sister confided in me about her husband's struggles, expressing, "I trust you and feel comfortable sharing these intimate details because you are honest, not because I fear judgment. But I'm troubled that his fear is starting to affect me." I replied, "Let's pray together." We both knelt and sought the Lord in prayer, and in that moment, we felt His presence and guidance.

175

I began the prayer by recalling 2 Timothy 1:7, which states, "For the Spirit God gave us does not make us timid, but gives us power, love, and self-discipline." I addressed the spirit of fear directly: "In the name of the Lord Jesus, I command you to leave this house and my brother; the Spirit God gave him is not one of fear, but of power and love. I command the spirit of fear that has taken root here to depart." I then turned to Psalm 23:4, proclaiming, "Though I walk through the valley of the shadow of death, I will fear no evil; for you are with me."

We continued praying, saying, "Lord, show this man daily that you are with him; increase his faith; let him lean on you, and as he does, may his fear vanish. You have told him repeatedly through your words, 'Do not be afraid, for I am with you.' Increase his faith so that he may confront his fears." God answered our prayer, and two weeks later, the individual experienced relief from the spirit of fear.

Fear is often described as a spirit. While it is natural to feel fear at times, we should not allow it to take hold of us. We are encouraged to commit everything to Jesus Christ and rely on His Word in our daily lives. As stated in Psalm 46:1-2: "God is our refuge and strength, an ever-present help in trouble. Therefore we will not fear, though the earth give way and the mountains fall into the heart of the sea."

For those tormented by fear, I encourage you to pray this prayer:

"Oh Lord, as your word says, 'Do not fear, for I am with you,' help me not to fear, for you are with me. Your word tells us, 'Do not be dismayed, for I am your God; I will strengthen you, help you, and hold you up with my right hand.' I commit my worries, hardships, and thoughts to you, trusting that you will uphold me just as you have promised. I trust you, my God, who assures me that you will never forsake or leave me. Thank you for your unwavering support. Amen."

I also pray for those who are being tormented by the spirit of fear. May God remove this spirit and fill you with peace. His comfort brings joy to the heart, providing both peace and love. Blessed be the name of our Lord Jesus forever.

In support of this, 2 Thessalonians 3:16 states, "Now may the Lord of peace himself give you peace at all times and in every way. The Lord be with all of you."

Chapter Fifteen

Serving With What Has Been Deposited Within Us

Everyone is unique in their own special way

Psalm 139:13-14 says, "You alone created my inner being. You knitted me together inside my mother. I will give thanks to you because I have been amazingly and miraculously made." God took the time to create each of us in a remarkable way. We are not all the same; some people are reserved, while others are outgoing. Some may be timid, and others may express their individuality through their clothing choices.

For example, some men embrace longer hairstyles, while some prefer preaching in jeans, while others choose to wear suits. Similarly, some women serve the Lord with makeup and stylish attire, while others prefer a more natural look. The Lord works through all of us. Our uniqueness can manifest in our dressing styles, manner of speaking, color preferences, choice of neighborhood, gait, laughter, and attitudes. Despite these differences, God has made each of us beautiful and wonderful.

It is not necessary for everyone to look or act the same; our diversity is part of God's design. No individual should be looked down upon for being different. We are called to accept and celebrate one another. The Lord embraces our uniqueness and encourages us to use it for His purpose. Discrimination against anyone based on their personality or choices is not right, as long as they do not harm others.

In many church communities, individuals who display uniqueness may struggle to find acceptance. There can be a tendency to believe that someone is not a genuine Christian unless they conform to certain behaviors, appearances, or ways of preaching that align with the majority. I have personally experienced negative comments such as, "Is this girl a genuine Christian? None of her things are Christian-like," simply because my expression of faith did not resemble that of others.

In some settings, only those who are reserved and quiet may be regarded as true Christians, leading to the rejection of those who are more expressive or different. This kind of discrimination should not be present; however, it does exist in various communities. On the contrary, there are churches that embrace diversity and actively assign individuals to roles that align with their unique gifts and personalities. For example, they might say, "You are friendly and enjoy greeting people, so you would be a great fit for the greeter position," or, "You have a talent for creativity; let's involve you in the creative team."

In my own experience, I was approached with a request to make announcements because I was told I had a pleasant voice. This opportunity allowed me to recognize my ability, even though it was clear that my voice was not suited for singing. The emphasis was on putting my strengths to use rather than trying to fit a conventional mold. I admire this approach and believe there is much to learn from communities that prioritize inclusion and appreciate the diverse gifts within their members.

I have encountered several young adults who possess significant potential for ministry but have not found opportunities to serve in the church. These individuals often go from home to home, sharing their faith and ministering to families. When I asked them why they haven't taken on roles within the church, they expressed that they feel excluded due to differences in appearance, style, and demeanor. They shared that their clothing, attitudes, or personal choices have been reasons for not being accepted. Such treatment should be reconsidered. Each person is uniquely created, and the talents and gifts given to us vary widely. As stated in Romans 12:6-8, "We have different gifts, according to the grace given to each of us. If your gift is prophesying, then prophesy in accordance with your faith; if it is serving, then serve; if it is teaching, then teach; if it is to encourage, then give encouragement; if it is giving, then give generously; if it is to lead, do it diligently; if it is to show mercy, do it cheerfully." This passage highlights the diversity of gifts and encourages individuals to use them in alignment with their faith.

Moreover, 1 Peter 4:11 emphasizes that everyone has a role to play: "If anyone speaks, they should do so as one who speaks the very words of God. If anyone serves, they should do so with the strength God provides, so that in all things God may be praised through Jesus Christ." Recognizing and embracing each person's unique contributions can lead to a more inclusive and vibrant community.

There was once a man known for his powerful prayer life; when he prayed, people felt blessed and transformed. One day, he was invited to preach and delivered an impactful sermon that resonated with many. After this experience, he declared, "From now on, I am not only a praying man but also a preacher." Initially, he was given a few opportunities to share sermons, but soon complaints arose. People expressed their desire for him to return to prayer, stating, "We came for prayer last Wednesday, but he was not present. We want him to pray for us."

When the pastor informed him of the congregation's preference for his presence at the prayer meetings, the man became irritated. He responded, "Why do you want to limit my ability to serve to just prayer? I have multiple gifts, and I don't want to confine myself to attending only the prayer meeting." His decision not to participate in the prayer meeting offended many who valued his prayer ministry. Subsequently, when he attempted to preach, interest in his sermons diminished.

This situation illustrates that when someone diverts from their primary calling, they may lose the unique impact they once had. Neglecting one's gifts can lead to a lack of fulfillment and support from the community. It is important to recognize that not everyone is called to preach or to sing; having a pleasant voice does not inherently qualify someone to be a singer. Others might excel in different roles, such as counseling or other forms of service. Embracing one's unique gifts and assignments is essential for finding true fulfillment and effectively contributing to the community.

Romans 12:6-8 highlights the diversity of gifts within the body of believers, stating, "If it is to encourage, then give encouragement; if it is giving, then give generously; if it is to lead, do it diligently; if it is to show mercy, do it cheerfully." This passage emphasizes the importance of recognizing and valuing the unique gifts that individuals possess. For instance, those who excel at counseling or exhortation bring invaluable support to others through their talents.

An illustrative example is a couple known for their generosity. They embrace their gift of giving and often remark, "Giving is our gift." Their commitment to supporting others—both in their community and beyond—has earned them a reputation as notable donors. By actively contributing to those in need, they have positively impacted many lives and have been described as having "set many individuals free from poverty." Their joyful approach to giving has not only led to personal blessings but has also cultivated a sense of community and gratitude among those they assist.

This couple's distinctive character stems from their willingness to embrace their gift of generosity, demonstrating that each individual's unique contributions play a vital role in the larger community.

The quote, "Don't be afraid of being different; be afraid of being the same as everyone else," attributed to Mehmet Meratidaw, further encourages individuals to embrace their uniqueness. It suggests that standing out can lead to clearer visibility and impact among crowds, reinforcing the idea that every person's distinct gifts can create a meaningful difference in the world around them.

In summary, recognizing and embracing one's unique gifts—whether in giving, counseling, or other areas—enriches both the individual and the community.

Since childhood, I have often felt different from others, which has led to experiences of discrimination. I recall instances where my dressing style and hairstyle were ridiculed. Even my sisters made fun of my hair, suggesting I should get it styled properly when they took me to a beauty salon, saying, "Get your disheveled hair done." For me, no hairstyle was as appealing as ruffled hair, yet they questioned my choices.

Throughout my life, I frequently encountered comments like, "You should not say such a thing; you should not do this; do not wear these clothes." As the pressure to conform intensified, I began to carve my own path. I remember modifying clothing I bought while in France, altering designs through cutting and sewing to suit my preferences. My friends in the faith laughed at these changes, but I remained unfazed. I have always recognized my differences, as many people have pointed out my unique dressing style and hairstyle.

I often reflected, "What is the problem as long as I do no harm to others and do not walk on the path of sin?"

Not everyone is expected to pursue careers like preaching, pastoring, singing, engineering, medicine, law, or aviation. When children express their future career aspirations, responses can vary. If a child says they want to become a hairdresser, fashion designer, dentist, firefighter, or electrician, parents might not always respond positively.

This can lead children to follow paths that align more with their parents' expectations rather than their own interests. Phrases like, "This isn't lucrative; why would you choose this when you have such potential?" can be discouraging, causing children to pursue careers that do not resonate with their true passions. As a result, they may lack engagement and effectiveness in their chosen fields because they are not following their natural gifts.

As previously mentioned, there are various gifts within the church and broader community. Each individual is endowed with unique talents, which can be utilized to benefit others. Sometimes, individuals may be unaware of their unique abilities, or they may hesitate to embrace them due to fear of non-acceptance. This hesitation can lead to underutilization of potential.

Encouraging individuals to recognize and pursue their unique gifts can foster both personal fulfillment and community growth.

We can effectively benefit others by utilizing the gifts that have been imparted to us. It's important to express gratitude for every talent you possess. Your gifts may include aspects of your personality, the ability to offer kind words, singing, decisiveness, generosity, preaching, wisdom, compassion, teaching skills, communication skills, or any area where you excel. It is wise to use these gifts to support others, as we are all members of one community. We should ensure that the gifts we have received do not go unused or overlooked.

The Lord has a specific purpose for each gift. During a Sunday school lesson, I encouraged my students to memorize this passage: "Not that we are sufficient of ourselves to think of anything as being from ourselves, but our sufficiency is from God."

I explained to them that God has crafted each of us uniquely; no two individuals are identical, and each of us has a distinct purpose. Being sufficient means doing everything possible with the gifts God has given us. For example, Joshua exemplified effective leadership by accomplishing the task of bringing down the fortified walls of Jericho through his abilities. He placed his trust in God and used his talents for a greater purpose.

This lesson was presented under the theme "Joshua, Who Tore Down the Walls of Jericho."

Joshua received clear instructions from God, and he diligently observed and obeyed those commands. I explained to the children, "The Lord commanded Joshua, and he followed those commands closely. God instructed Joshua to take the town, and he shared these instructions with his people to focus their attention on God. The Lord directed Joshua to march around the city's walls for seven days, and Joshua organized his army, including seven priests." I encouraged them to read Joshua 6:1-26 to see how the story unfolds. "Joshua was effective in his leadership because he allowed God to guide him and followed His instructions. We, too, can utilize the gifts given to us in a similar way."

I emphasized the importance of being thankful for our talents and abilities and using them to serve God by serving others. By doing so, we can become trustworthy friends and leaders. To help emphasize this, I asked the children to list at least five things they could do during the week. We discussed how one of these goals could be directed toward helping someone else. For instance, if someone excels in school, they might assist a peer who is struggling; if they have singing skills, they could lead a worship session; if they are good at sports, they can help others improve their skills; and if they are artistic, they could create drawings to uplift others. I shared these examples to illustrate how we can recognize our gifts and use them to help others, just as these children can do.

Teaching children is a gift I cherish, and I find joy in working with those aged 5 through 12. In preparation for my Sunday school class, I dedicate time throughout the week to plan my lessons and pray for guidance, asking, "Lord, let me find favor in the eyes of these children." I believe we can achieve success when we serve using the gifts that the Lord has given us, making prayer and intentional use of our talents a priority.

It is important to honor the gifts we have received, no matter how small they may seem. By being faithful with these gifts and committing ourselves fully, we may be called to greater responsibilities and receive even more blessings.

I have observed individuals who naturally attract others simply by being themselves. One such person in my church is a girl who is well-loved by everyone. She shows affection to all, helps those in need, and takes care of children from various families. Her cheerful demeanor endears her to the community; people often feel comfortable visiting her home spontaneously. Her presence brings a sense of warmth, and it is common for visitors to bring gifts for her children out of appreciation for her kindness. She also makes a point to care for those who are unwell by bringing food when she visits them.

One day at church, a preacher spoke about spiritual gifts. After the sermon, a woman approached me and expressed her feelings of inadequacy, saying, "I do not have any gift; my time is running out, and I still don't know what my gift is." I responded with a laugh, telling her, "Is there anyone as gifted as you? You have served by comforting others, supporting them, showing love, reconciling differences, and listening. Those are unique gifts—characteristics of Jesus himself. It's not necessary to deliver a sermon from a pulpit to have a significant impact. I've never seen anyone with a gift quite like yours; it's both large and unique, and you benefit many people." She was moved to tears and replied, "You say this because you love me." I reassured her, "Everyone loves you." She then asked, "So, is this a gift?" and I affirmed, "It is indeed a significant gift."

When she passed away at a young age due to cancer, many people mourned her loss. Her funeral was attended by a diverse crowd—men, women, individuals from various backgrounds, including black, white, Muslim, Orthodox,

Catholic, Protestant, Filipinos, and Chinese. This turnout reflected the many lives she had positively influenced during her time on earth.

I often think about the woman who cleaned the toilets at the church. Every Sunday, she arrived dressed neatly, changed into cleaning clothes, and put on gloves to tackle the task at hand, doing so with a smile and without any payment. One day, I approached her to express my observation. I said, "I often see you cleaning the toilets, and you seem to do it happily." She responded, "I feel glad because I am serving the Lord and His people. Service doesn't always need to be visible; even if people don't see or thank you, the Lord does. Whatever you do, do it as a service to the Lord; if you serve Him with the little you have, He will put you in charge of more."

She went on to explain her perspective, saying, "I feel happy when a toilet is clean, just as I feel happy when my own home is tidy. If I find joy in cleaning my house, how could I not feel the same way about the house of God?" I thanked her for her dedication, and she replied, "When you start with the little God has given you, He ensures that you reach a higher level. What I am doing may not seem significant to others, and some might even laugh, but I have a reward from the Lord." Hearing her words brought tears to my eyes, and I said, "How fortunate you are!" Her lesson on humility and service is one I will carry with me always.

This sister serves God by preaching the word, and the Lord is using her in remarkable ways. She has found favor with both God and people. Many believers visit her home, asking for prayer, and she never seems to tired, even if she prays day and night.

The Holy Spirit has granted her great grace.

Though she may appear ordinary and may not be widely recognized by many, the Lord knows who she is. She has embraced the gift the Lord has given her and has become an example for others. The Lord lifts up those who honor Him, and this sister has served Him with sincerity. The Lord has considered her dedication and has ensured that she has everything she needs. She experiences abundant joy and peace.

However, this is not always the case in our community.

Often, people desire to serve in ways that draw attention and recognition from others. Some have questioned, "How long will you teach children? Will you be teaching them for the rest of your life?" What they may not understand is that teaching children is a meaningful ministry for me. It brings me joy to help them develop a love for Jesus Christ by sharing His story: His role as a healer, His greatness, goodness, mercy, kindness, generosity, fatherhood, protective nature, and faithfulness. Serving children brings me a sense of fulfillment that few other things can match.

My joy comes from seeing Jesus exalted and worshipped by both children and adults. This is my primary goal. I have taught many children, and among their parents, only three have regularly expressed their gratitude to me. I remember one parent, named Koni, who frequently thanked and blessed me. However, I focused on my enjoyment of the work and my dedication to serving the Lord rather than seeking recognition.

It is easy to feel overlooked when serving in small ways, as often our contributions go unnoticed. Yet, when we understand that our efforts are for the Lord and that there is a reward awaiting us, our hearts can remain filled with hope rather than despair.

Therefore, when we do what we do for the Lord, we can protect our hearts from discouragement. It is important to approach our tasks with love and joy, and above all, to do everything for the glory of the Lord Jesus Christ, as stated in Colossians 3:17: "And whatever you do, whether in word or deed, do it all in the name of the Lord Jesus, giving thanks to God the Father through Him."

It is true that we may sometimes feel unappreciated when our efforts seem undervalued. I have experienced this feeling multiple times and have faced various challenges. I regularly bring these challenges to the Lord, placing them at His feet and moving forward. I choose not to dwell on negative thoughts, as I trust that the Lord has a purpose for me.

Embrace the Joy of Serving

Serving others can be a source of tremendous joy, and it's important to focus on that joy regardless of whether our efforts are acknowledged. When we engage in service, we often find fulfillment in the act itself, knowing that we are contributing to the well-being of others and aligning with a greater purpose.

By framing our experiences positively, we can cultivate an attitude of gratitude and appreciation for the opportunities we have to make a difference. Each interaction, each lesson taught, and each moment spent in service can be seen as a chance to express love and compassion, benefiting both the giver and the recipient.

In the journey of serving, there may be times when recognition is scarce. However, it is essential to remember that the impact of our service can extend far beyond what is visible. The joy derived from serving others is rooted in the knowledge that we are part of something meaningful.

Embracing this perspective allows us to focus on the intrinsic rewards of service—the connections made, the lives touched, and the personal growth experienced. Ultimately, the act of serving can become a profound joy in itself, enriching our own lives while fostering a spirit of community and support among those we serve.

Chapter Sixteen

Let Us Get Encouraged

The scripture in 1 Thessalonians 5:11 states, "Therefore encourage one another and build each other up, just as in fact you are doing." This verse highlights the importance of supporting and uplifting one another in our daily lives.

In 1 Thessalonians 5:14-15, we are advised to be proactive in our relationships: "And we urge you, brothers and sisters, warn those who are idle and disruptive, encourage the disheartened, help the weak, be patient with everyone. Make sure that nobody pays back wrong for wrong, but always strive to do what is good for each other and for everyone else." This passage underscores the need for compassion, patience, and resilience in our interactions.

Colossians 3:16 further reinforces this idea: "Let the word of Christ dwell in you richly in all wisdom, teaching and admonishing one another in psalms and hymns and spiritual songs, singing with grace in your hearts to the Lord." This verse suggests that sharing uplifting messages through various forms of expression can enrich our communal experience.

Hebrews 10:25 encourages regular connection: "Let us not give up meeting together, as some are in the habit of doing, but encouraging one another—and all the more as you see the Day approaching." This emphasizes the value of community and the support that comes from mutual encouragement.

Lastly, 1 Peter 4:8 reminds us of the foundational role of love: "Above all, love each other deeply, because love covers over a multitude of sins." This message speaks to the importance of fostering an atmosphere of love and understanding.

As we reflect on these teachings, may we commit to becoming sources of encouragement within our communities. By fostering a supportive environment, we can help one another navigate challenges and promote a sense of belonging.

Our Bible encourages us to uplift one another through the teachings of the Lord. The apostle Paul, in Philippians 1:3-5, expresses his gratitude: "I thank my God every time I remember you. In all my prayers for all of you, I always pray with joy because of your partnership in the gospel from the first day until now."

Paul's words reflect his deep appreciation for the people he is addressing. He shares that he prays for them with joy. While our service is ultimately to the Lord and we may not seek recognition from others, encouraging and uplifting one another can lead to increased joy and motivation. Such encouragement fosters love, humility, and a joyful spirit in all involved.

I personally express gratitude for the kindness shown to me, often sharing my thanks on social media with my sisters. Though some have suggested that I should express my appreciation in private, I find joy in publicly acknowledge-ing their support. I have come to realize the positive impact of encouraging and thanking individuals in front of others.

Timothy was a young minister of God, and the apostle Paul expressed gratitude to the believers in Christ by saying, "We ought always to thank God for you, brothers and sisters, and rightly so, because your faith is growing more and more, and the love all of you have for one another is increasing."

When we focus on the phrase "We ought always to thank God for you," it highlights the importance of thanking and encouraging one another as an obligation. Paul recognized the benefits of expressing gratitude, understanding that it fosters a stronger sense of community and love.

Thanking and encouraging one another can indeed enhance love within a community. Paul, while in prison, wrote several letters to encourage the believers, consistently emphasizing his prayers and thanksgiving for them.

In 2 Thessalonians 1:11-12, Paul states: "With this in mind, we constantly pray for you, that our God may make you worthy of his calling, and that by his power he may bring to fruition your every desire for goodness and your every deed prompted by faith. We pray this so that the name of our Lord Jesus may be glorified in you, and you in him, according to the grace of our God and the Lord Jesus Christ."

In Numbers 6:24-26, God conveys a message to Moses about blessing the Israelites, instructing Aaron and his sons with the words: "The Lord bless you and keep you; the Lord make his face shine on you and be gracious to you; the Lord turn his face toward you and give you peace." God emphasizes the importance of this blessing, stating that through it, His name will be placed on the Israelites, and He will bless them.

This message reflects the deep comfort and strength that such words of blessing can provide. God understood the significance of encouraging His people, recognizing that regularly sharing these words of comfort with friends and family can have a profound impact.

Furthermore, it is important to support, comfort, and express gratitude to one another, especially those who serve in the church. While they may dedicate their work to the Lord, encouragement and prayers from the community are vital to their well-being. Unfortunately, this kind of support may not always be as visible as it should be.

It's important to recognize that the attitude within the church can significantly impact the overall community. Often, there may exist a perception that those who serve—whether laypeople or ministers—do so solely for the Lord, which can lead to a lack of acknowledgment and support for their efforts. This oversight can result in feelings of sadness and disconnect when individuals who have faithfully served choose to leave or distance themselves from the church.

Every person who serves in the church deserves appreciation and attention. Simple acts such as thanking them and inquiring about their well-being can foster a sense of belonging and encouragement. It's crucial that church leaders actively promote a culture of support and mutual comfort among all congregants.

God's instruction to Moses to bless the Israelites underscores the importance of uplifting one another. As followers of God, we are called to bless and express gratitude toward His children. The health of the church community depends on genuine cooperation and encouragement, built on love.

Additionally, it is concerning when pride or conceit manifests within church settings, as it can hinder the spirit of unity and fellowship. While such attitudes may exist in any community, it is essential for those who profess to follow the teachings of Christ to embody His character by demonstrating love, support, and humility toward each other.

Ultimately, mutual encouragement and recognition are vital in building a strong and vibrant church community, allowing all members to thrive and grow in their faith together.

Naomi speaks a comforting and encouraging word to her daughters-in-law, which brings them to weep loudly. Similarly, Boaz offers an encouraging word to Ruth, saying, "May the Lord repay you for what you have done. May you be richly rewarded by the Lord, the God of Israel, under whose wings you have come to take refuge."

In response, Ruth says, "May I continue to find favor in your eyes, my lord. You have put me at ease by speaking kindly to your servant—though I do not have the standing of one of your servants." This exchange in Ruth 2:19 illustrates how Naomi edifies her daughters-in-law and Boaz comforts Ruth. Ruth expresses that Boaz has brought her comfort, despite her lower status as a gleaner.

Boaz's gratitude and kindness towards Ruth are significant, as he could have simply regarded her as an employee and felt no obligation to thank or comfort her. Nevertheless, he chooses to do so because he is a decent man, reflecting the attributes of God. Ruth, in turn, feels greatly comforted by his words.

This narrative teaches us a valuable lesson about kindness and respect within relationships, regardless of status or position.

Though I am paid for my work, my boss consistently checks in with me by asking, "How are you? Are you doing well? Is anything lacking? What can I do to help?" When he needs me to substitute for an employee who is absent, he writes me a note using thoughtful language. If I respond with, "I cannot," he lightens the mood by sending a sad face symbol. Conversely, if I reply, "Yes," he responds with a smiley face symbol, a joke, or an uplifting word. He is my boss and could simply give instructions without this additional communication; however, he chooses to foster a supportive environment where we encourage one another. If someone asks, "Who have we learned this from?" the answer is our boss.

He advises us to always encourage each other, and he leads by example through his own encouragement.

In 2 Samuel 2:5-6, we see David expressing gratitude to those who buried Saul, despite their complicated relationship. David acknowledges the kindness of those who buried Saul, saying, "The Lord bless you for showing this kindness to Saul your master by burying him. May the Lord now show you kindness and faithfulness, and I too will show you the same favor because you have done this." We see David bless and encourage those who buried Saul; it is difficult to find such individuals today. Many struggle to treat even those close to them with love, let alone to bless those who have persecuted them. David did not express relief that his pursuer had died; instead, he thanked and blessed those who buried him. This reflects the nature of Jesus and illustrates how we should conduct ourselves when His presence is evident in our lives.

In Romans 1:7-8, the Apostle Paul states, "Grace and peace to you from God our Father and from the Lord Jesus Christ.

First, I thank my God through Jesus Christ for all of you, because your faith is being reported all over the world." Here, Paul expresses gratitude for the Roman believers, acknowledging that their faith has had a significant impact. Similarly, in 1 Thessalonians 1:2-3, Paul comforts and encourages the believers in Thessalonica, saying, "We always thank God for all of you and continually mention you in our prayers. We remember before our God and Father your work produced by faith, your labor prompted by love, and your endurance inspired by hope in our Lord Jesus Christ."

These passages emphasize the importance of gratitude and encouragement in building community and fostering spiritual growth.

In this passage, the Apostle Paul emphasizes the importance of gratitude when he writes, "We always thank God for all of you," rather than saying "we sometimes thank God." He makes it clear that he consistently prays for the Thessalonian believers. Despite their suffering, these individuals joyfully preached the word, encouraged by Paul's presence and support. Their faith became an example to other believers in Macedonia and beyond, demonstrating the impact of their unwavering trust in God.

The Thessalonian believers not only experienced Paul's encouragement but also became a blessing to others because of it. This reinforces the call for all of us to encourage and comfort one another, rather than taking advantage of others. It is essential for congregants to thank and uplift their pastors and church leaders. Well-known figures in ministry, including singers and preachers, also require encouragement and support; being in the public eye does not shield them from the need for affirmation and prayer.

In 1 Samuel 30:6, we find that "David found strength in the Lord his God." This serves as a reminder for us not to neglect our spiritual well-being during challenging times. Even when faced with adversity, as David was when the people turned against him, he sought strength in God instead of succumbing to despair. David did not dwell on why he was in such a predicament; rather, he chose to reinforce his faith. There is much to learn from David's example as we navigate our own challenges.

Many disheartening things have happened to me in the past. I have experienced isolation, and disdain, and I have felt profound loneliness. There is little that I have not faced; what I write to you reflects my own experiences. In moments of darkness and despair, I turn to the Word of the Lord. The Lord always comforts me. When I read the scriptures, I am reminded that Jesus endured suffering much like I have. He was despised, isolated, insulted, and spat upon; yet, he did not waver from his purpose.

Many people have faced significant challenges in their lives. They have overcome their adversities by strengthening themselves in the Lord and entrusting their burdens to Him. Satan seeks to lead us to neglect ourselves and to lose hope in the Lord. However, we can discern the works and thoughts of Satan; by setting aside his lies and finding strength and comfort in the Word of the Lord, we can ultimately overcome and triumph over these challenges.

In the past, I shared my problems with others, hoping they would help me find solutions. Yet, I remember one individual telling me, "You always talk about problems; ask the Lord why this is happening to you. Perhaps there is a curse in your life." On another occasion, someone remarked, "I came to this country after you, but look how my quality of life has improved." This experience has taught me that while some people offer truth and comfort, others may take pleasure in others' difficulties. Therefore, it's important to be cautious about whom we confide in.

Throughout my life, I have learned that only Jesus is truly trustworthy. He has consistently demonstrated His faithfuless to me. In moments of pain, I have learned to share my problems and secrets with the Lord. I turn to Jesus Christ, casting all my cares upon Him, as He knows how to guide me. He does not judge or disparage me; I trust Him completely. I encourage others to commit their worries and concerns to the Lord.

Instead of dwelling on our troubles, we should find comfort in the Word of God and keep moving forward. With Jesus by our side, we can find sufficiency and support.

Every individual faces their own struggles. I have seen people who have neglected their well-being, and some have even taken their own lives due to their problems.

Absolutely! Encouraging one another is vital for building support and resilience in our lives. Here are a few ways we can inspire and uplift each other:

1. Sharing Stories: When we share our experiences and how we've overcome challenges, it can provide hope to others facing similar issues. Personal stories of resilience remind us that we are not alone.

2. Active Listening: Sometimes, simply listening to someone can offer them the comfort they need. Being present and validating their feelings can be incredibly encouraging.

3. Affirming Positivity: Complimenting each other on our strengths and achievements, no matter how small, can boost morale. Recognizing the good in ourselves and others fosters a positive environment.

4. Offering Support: Letting someone know you're there for them, whether through words of encouragement or practical help, can make a significant difference.

5. Encouraging Self-Care: Reminding one another to take time for self-care and prioritize mental health is essential. It's important to be gentle with ourselves and each other.

6. Prayer and Reflection: For those who are spiritual, praying for one another or reflecting on positive scripture can be a source of great comfort and strength.

You might wonder, "Why?" This question arises when someone they trusted betrays them or when a confidant reveals their secrets. When faced with judgment from others, they may fall into despair and begin to engage in unhealthy behaviors.

Once, I spoke with a young woman who was both beautiful and bright, yet I found myself confused by the way she had neglected her well-being. Concerned, I asked, "What has happened to you?" She replied, "I am fine." I offered her my phone number, saying, "You can call me anytime." I don't like to trouble others, and because she was such a promising individual, I wanted to help prevent her future from being derailed.

For two months, she didn't call. I would occasionally see her around, but it wasn't until two months later that she reached out. She said, "I am ready now; I can tell you everything. But first, I need some money to buy a cigarette." I responded, "We can discuss the cigarette when we meet." She insisted, "I can't talk without smoking first; so it's not possible for us to meet." I reiterated, "We can talk about cigarettes when we meet." She agreed and eventually came to see me.

Interestingly, when she arrived, she didn't mention the cigarette. After greeting me, she immediately began to share her story.

After turning 18, my attraction to men declined, and I found myself loving women instead. I resisted this feeling for a long time, but it persisted. Eventually, I began dating women. However, since this was uncommon in my community, I kept it a secret. My parents never suspected anything until one day, my father caught me. He then told my mother and brothers about it; they insulted me and chased me out of the house, telling me I should never come to church again.

My father wept profusely, saying tearfully, "Lord, what have I done to deserve this? How have I offended you? This child I raised in the church is corrupted." That night, I contemplated ending my life. A sister who was close to me comforted me, and I decided against it.

One day, while I was smoking a cigarette with a sister on the road, some individuals approached us. They spat at me and said, "What are you doing? You will end up in hell." They judged me harshly, labeling me as indecent and a reproach, uttering, "May the Lord forgive you."

There was no one who encouraged me or said, "I will pray for you." Whether believers or non-believers, people often condemned me. This constant judgment made me hate going to church.

Despite this, I prayed with a friend, and she began to attend the church where I go. She even started bringing her friends along. My friend is no longer in her previous difficult situation; she has moved to another city for work.

When someone shares their struggles with you, it's important not to judge them immediately. Instead, offer support, handle their issues with care, and keep their secrets. The Lord can change that person, and we should be patient with them.

Everyone who comes to church carries their own questions and struggles. They need someone who will embrace, comfort, uplift, correct, and support them. No one wants to experience the isolation they may have felt in the world, especially in a place meant for community. Many individuals have lost hope for various reasons and choose to stay home instead of going to church, rationalizing, "What difference will it make if I go?" However, this mindset does not solve their problems. The enemy seeks to instill despair in our hearts; we must be aware of this.

For those who have chosen to stay home because of feelings of isolation and hopelessness, take heart—Jesus is with you. Find comfort in the word of the Lord; remember that Jesus will never forsake you. Do not pay attention to the lies of despair. If you have stopped attending church, consider reaching out to your pastors for prayer and counseling support.

As stated in 2 Corinthians 1:4, "He comforts us in all our troubles, so that we can comfort those in any trouble with the comfort we ourselves receive from God."

We can only help others if we take the time to comfort and strengthen ourselves. Had I allowed despair to overwhelm me during my own struggles, I would not be writing this book today. There were many moments when I felt hopeless, and I even contemplated taking my own life. Yet the Lord intervened, saying, "No." He lifted me from my despair, affirming, "Wongel, I have a purpose for you." I am grateful for where I am now, and I give thanks to God for guiding me through.

Chapter Seventeen

The Lord Who Does Not See the Way Humans Do

Lift People UP Do Not Put Them Down

It troubles me to observe how some individuals disparage and harbor animosity toward others. Comments such as "He is not educated" or "I do not like this person" can rob us of our peace. I do not see any attributes of the Lord in such behavior. It is not the nature of Jesus to belittle or cause others to stumble but to uplift and edify them.

Since childhood, I have recognized that those who are despised often receive favor from God. I have experienced being looked down upon by some, yet I also feel deeply loved by the Lord. Regardless of whether I am at work or elsewhere, He has granted me favor in the eyes of children, the elderly, and the youth. They always express joy in my presence, wanting to be near me—not because of my appearance, but because of my cheerfulness. They have told me, "We feel happy when we are with you." I share this not out of arrogance, but to highlight the work of the Lord in my life.

I visit the gym four times a week for physical exercise, where I encountered a girl who is deaf and has limited mobility. Despite her challenges, she never loses hope and consistently comes to the gym. We became friends, and her joy is evident when she sees me. My only contribution has been to greet her with a smile and embrace her warmly. Although she cannot speak, the sounds she makes in joy and her determination to call my name are truly remarkable.

Her mother approached me and remarked, "She feels joyful when she sees you, but I do not understand why. I have never seen her so happy. Could you spend a few minutes with her twice a week? I would be willing to pay for your time." I felt tears welling in my eyes as I thanked the Lord for the favor I found in this girl. I responded to her mother, "Every time I come to the gym, I will dedicate 10 minutes to her at no charge." Her mother was very pleased, and my joy was immeasurable.

This is a significant moment for me, as the girl I befriended brought along her friends who are also deaf and have disabilities. We spend valuable time together, and it was a heartwarming experience.

It's important to recognize that some of us may have grown up in difficult environments, perhaps facing abuse or verbal insults from family members or others. Such experiences can lead to feelings of inferiority and a sense of being trapped in a cycle of negative expectations for the future.

However, it's crucial to reflect on the stories of individuals like Jephthah and Joseph, who overcame their circumstances.

God often works through those who are marginalized, rejected, or looked down upon. I recall a powerful story shared with me by someone who faced significant challenges:

"My mother is struggling financially, and my father has a problem with alcohol. My mother constantly tells me, 'It would have been better if you were never born; you are worthless; bringing you into this world was a mistake.' Growing up with these words haunted me. I became resentful and eventually ran away from home. Now, as an adult, I can't escape the impact of her words. I find it hard to form friendships; I've had various friends but have cut ties with them for no obvious reason. I become frustrated over trivial matters and can't hold onto a job for long."

Hearing his story brought me to tears. I asked him, "Is your mother still alive?" He replied, "Yes, but I haven't spoken to her and don't want to see her." I suggested to him,

"The first step you should take is to approach your mother and seek peace with her. Ask for her forgiveness, and be willing to forgive her as well. Only then will you find healing, and the Lord can begin to work in your life."

He asked, "In my life?"

I affirmed, "Yes."

He then stated, "I don't even know who Jesus is; I do not go to church; I do not have a religion." I responded, "Jesus loves you; He knows you even if you do not know Him." He inquired, "Where can I find this Lord then?" I replied, "Right here," and I prayed for him. He accepted the Lord Jesus Christ as his personal savior and asked his mother for forgiveness. His mother was deeply moved. He began supporting both his mother and father, and ultimately, they also came to believe that Jesus is the only savior and started serving Him. They have a large family, and he mentioned, "Many people come to our house for prayer." I was truly amazed by the work being done.

Had I not encouraged and prayed for this individual, it is unlikely he would have sought forgiveness from his mother or accepted the Lord. It is evident that the Lord uplifts those who are marginalized.

He works through individuals in various circumstances. Jesus loves you and invites you to serve Him.

Once, I was standing in line at a bank for a transaction when I noticed that one of the tellers had a speech impediment.

The woman in front of me turned to me and said, "How do they assign the responsibilities of a teller to a person with a speech impediment?" I chose not to reply and continued waiting for my turn. She then added, "I do not want to go to her; if I am assigned to her, I will let you go ahead of me." I simply responded, "Yes."

The teller with the speech impediment worked more briskly than the other tellers, which helped move the queue along quickly. Eventually, the lady before me was assigned to her. As she did not want to go to this teller, she told me, "You go ahead of me; I will go to another teller." I agreed and proceeded to the teller.

Since the teller completed my financial transaction in just a few moments, the woman who had initially been in front of me found herself assigned to the same teller again. However, she chose to let the person behind her in line go ahead of her before approaching the teller.

As I continued to observe the situation at the bank, the same lady found herself assigned to the teller for the third time. This time, instead of deferring to another person in line, she approached the teller directly, despite her initial reservations. I remained curious about how this encounter would unfold.

The teller efficiently processed the woman's transaction in just a few minutes. Afterward, the woman approached me, and I remarked, "Is she not lovable?" To my surprise, she responded with, "She is amazing." She pointed out the badge the teller was wearing, revealing that she was actually the manager of the bank.

This experience serves as a powerful reminder: it's important not to judge a person based on outward appearances. The Lord works through everyone and can use each individual's unique qualities to contribute positively to their surroundings.

What I see nowadays is quite confusing. Instead of comforting individuals and saying, "I will help you as much as I can," we often demean others. We do not seem to feel any embarrassment when we label someone with phrases like, "He is not educated," or "She is this kind of person." We create our own standards and use them to categorize individuals. Once someone is placed into a specific category, we often expect them to remain there. This reality saddens me.

The Lord has made us all different, yet we may look down on those who are unlike us, whether due to lower status, lack of eloquence in prayer and preaching, education level, cleanliness, or intelligence. However, this should not be the case. I once read a quote: "When we label people and put them in different boxes, we do not see them for who they truly are." The Lord often works through those who are least expected and who may be despised by others. This was true for Peter and John.

Peter and John were considered uneducated and ordinary individuals, often looked down upon by others. Their circumstances led the Pharisees, the High Priest, and the elders to categorize them as incapable of making significant contributions. However, Jesus frequently worked through those whom society regarded as despised or overlooked, surprising many.

The transformation that occurred in the lives of Peter and John left others astonished. The Scriptures note that they were genuinely amazed by the remarkable changes brought about by Jesus in these individuals. This serves as a reminder that Jesus does not judge based on societal standards; rather, He can work wonders in the lives of those whom others might dismiss.

It is disheartening to see that some among us in the Habesha community often say, "My ethnicity is better than yours; I am better than you." This rivalry should not even exist. However, the Lord continues to work through those who are marginalized. The challenges faced by individuals like

Paul, Peter, and John were significant. In reference to this, Paul writes, "We are hard-pressed on every side, yet not crushed; we are perplexed, but not in despair; persecuted, but not forsaken; struck down, but not destroyed."

It's indeed a complex and often painful issue when divisions arise within communities based on ethnicity or other identities. The sentiment of competing superiority can create tension and discord, detracting from the unity that individuals should strive for. It's essential to recognize that value is not inherent in one's ethnicity or status; rather, it lies in one's character, actions, and how they treat others.

Ultimately, fostering a spirit of acceptance and love, regardless of differences, can lead to a more harmonious community. It's essential to focus on what unites rather than divides, recognizing that everyone has unique contributions to make.

The Lord loves everyone and often works through those who are overlooked or least expected. I remember experiencing this deeply when I was just 12 years old; my name became well-known in my neighborhood, and some people came to me asking for prayer. During this time, I was blessed with the gifts of knowledge and healing. Some individuals who visited my home to seek prayer would laugh and ask, "Are you Wongel? Are you the one praying for us?" They did not take me seriously. However, I was unaware of how the Spirit of the Lord transformed me during those moments of prayer.

I have a profound love for prayer. When I closed my bedroom door behind me, I often lost track of time while in prayer. The presence of the Lord filled my space, bringing me great joy. I felt that the Lord called me at a young age, and whenever I knelt down to pray, I sensed His presence enveloping me. It was truly remarkable how the Lord used me during that time.

Many years later, during a prayer meeting in Toronto, Canada, I experienced the Lord's presence once again—a presence I had become accustomed to since my childhood. It was an indescribable experience, and at times, we found ourselves praying until dawn without realizing how much time had passed. On one occasion, a woman approached me and said, "How the Lord loves you! I saw a very tall man clothed in white standing beside you, accompanied by many angels. I was surprised to see this because I had never considered that the Lord would work through you. I tell you this: The Lord loves you so much. Please forgive me for having looked down on you."

I had not previously known this woman; she was invited by someone else to the prayer meeting and had only seen me for the second time that day. On her first encounter with me, she had felt a sense of contempt. However, it is evident that the Lord often works through those who are overlooked or despised. I frequently hear of individuals forsaking, belittling, or disparaging one another, but the Lord continuously focuses on those who are marginalized.

I have a deep love for worshipping the Lord. When I engage in worship, the Spirit of the Lord comes upon me in a way that I cannot control, and sometimes I feel as though I am being taken up into heaven. It is truly indescribable. However, many people do not comprehend my experience.

Once, a woman approached me and said, "I feel joyful when I see you worshipping the Lord, and I often find myself envious of you." She went on to mention, "My husband watched you give a testimony last week, and he was surprised by what you shared. He said, 'I did not think Wongel knew the word of God; I only saw her as someone who was good at wearing fancy clothes.' But the Lord spoke to him, and he felt ashamed. It's not right to categorize someone without evidence."

I was somewhat taken aback by her husband's previous characterization of me, so I responded, "Please tell your husband that I am more than just someone who wears nice clothes; I am a beloved child of the Lord Jesus and His minister. While I may appear to you as someone focused on 'fashionable' attire, I am a woman who stands with Jesus by my side." She laughed and replied, "He knows this; what I told you was his opinion from the past. I would prefer to ask him to apologize to you."

It's important to address the misconceptions that some people have about my character and responsibilities. I sometimes hear remarks like, "Are you such a responsible woman? We didn't expect that given that you are often seen with children." Others might say, "Since we always see you laughing and playing, we didn't think you knew the Lord properly." To these comments, I respond, "I am cheerful because I have Jesus, who is my peace and fills my heart with joy."

Unfortunately, it's common to encounter attitudes of disdain or condescension toward others, which should be challenged and brought to an end. Disparaging one ethnicity while elevating another is particularly harmful and should be unequivocally condemned. Such attitudes benefit no one. We are all created from one humanity; none of us chooses the lineage into which we are born. Disrespecting those whom God has created is not aligned with His teachings.

What we need to understand is that we don't find God in perfection—since no one is perfect—but rather in our humanity and imperfections. Our faith is inspired by the understanding that God called individuals like Moses and the disciples, despite their flaws and limitations. The good news is that God knows our abilities and still invites us to share His grace and love with others in the world.

It's a powerful reminder that God can work through anyone, regardless of their imperfections or circumstances. Throughout history, we've seen examples like David, Gideon, and Moses, who were called by God despite facing various challenges and feelings of inadequacy.

Gideon's story is particularly compelling. He was hiding from the Midianites when God called him while he was threshing wheat in a winepress, a setting that reflects his fear and vulnerability. Yet, the angel addressed him as "O mighty man of valor," highlighting that God's perspective often transcends our own view of ourselves. It serves as an encouragement to recognize the potential within ourselves, even when we feel least deserving or capable.

This narrative illustrates that God's grace and purpose can shine through our weaknesses and that He often chooses those who feel overlooked or undervalued to accomplish His work. It's important for individuals to honor their own intrinsic worth and abilities, remembering that everyone has a role to play in the greater narrative of grace and love.

God is capable of working through even the most imperfect and unexpected individuals, just like you and me. Since the beginning of time, He has used those who may seem unlikely to reveal His perfect grace and love.

God can be found in nearly everyone, including you and me. He used David, who was looked down upon, and Gideon, who felt despised because he was "the youngest in his family." He also used Moses. The work of the Lord continues to amaze me.

It's important to highlight certain aspects of Gideon's story. When God called him, Gideon was hiding from the Midianites, threshing wheat in a winepress. Despite his fear and trembling, the angel of the Lord addressed him with the words, "The LORD is with you, O mighty man of valor." This highlights that God does not view our weaknesses and limitations in the same way we do; instead, He sees beyond them. He referred to the frightened man as "a mighty man of valor."

I feel saddened when individuals belittle themselves or fail to recognize the strength that lies within them. God consistently works through those who are broken, marginalized, and least expected to fulfill His purpose. When Gideon was called, he replied, "My clan is the weakest in Manasseh, and I am the least in my father's house" (Judges 6:12-15).

Although Gideon despised himself, God assured him that He would demonstrate His might through his weakness. God said to Gideon, "Surely I will be with you, and you shall strike the Midianites as one man." The story that follows recounts Gideon's victory over the Midianites, highlighting God's tendency to focus on those who are often despised.

I recall attending a conference at the Dayspring Retreat Center after a sister in the Lord insisted that I accompany her. Various pastors from different countries delivered inspiring sermons, making it a wonderful experience. On the final day of the conference, we were told that a 19-year-old pastor from Paris would pray for us. As he began to pray, he repeatedly declared, "Lord, you are wonderful; you surpass our understanding."

As he continued, the atmosphere shifted, and soon everyone began speaking in tongues. Many were deeply touched by the Spirit of God, and some fell to the ground. The presence of God filled the room. My companion and I found ourselves immersed in this divine experience, completely unaware of our surroundings. It was palpable that the Spirit of God was moving powerfully through the assembly, touching every individual present.

That day, I felt an intensity of the Holy Spirit's presence like never before, affecting everyone from the youngest to the oldest among us. Interestingly, this young pastor did not lay hands on anyone or physically touch anyone; he could only speak limited English. Despite not being known to anyone in the congregation, God used him in a remarkable way. When the program concluded, a line formed as everyone, without exception, wanted to hug and congratulate him. It was a testament to how the Lord often works through those who are not anticipated or recognized.

Throughout history, there have been many instances where individuals perceived as unlikely or overlooked have defied expectations and achieved great success. These are often individuals whom others may have doubted or even given up on, including their own families. Their stories highlight the potential for resilience, determination, and talent to lead to significant accomplishments, regardless of initial circumstances. Such examples serve as a reminder that everyone has the capacity to make a meaningful impact, often surprising those who underestimate them.

Here are some individuals who were overlooked or faced significant challenges but went on to achieve great success:

1. J.K. Rowling - Before the success of the Harry Potter series, Rowling faced multiple rejections from publishers and struggled with personal hardships, including financial difficulties as a single mother.

2. Oprah Winfrey - Overcoming a troubled childhood marked by poverty and abuse, Oprah became a media mogul and one of the most influential women in the world.

3. Albert Einstein - Initially considered a poor student and thought to have learning difficulties, Einstein went on to become one of the most renowned physicists in history.

4. Steve Jobs - After being removed from the company he co-founded, Jobs went on to create products and innovations that revolutionized technology and design.

5. Maya Angelou - Despite experiencing trauma and discrimination throughout her early life, Angelou became a celebrated author, poet, and activist whose work has inspired many.

6. Walt Disney - Facing multiple job rejections and several failed business ventures, Disney eventually created an

entertainment empire known for innovation in animation and theme parks.

7. Thomas Edison - Often labeled as a poor student and told he would never amount to much, Edison became one of the most famous inventors in history, holding over a thousand patents.

8. Nicolas Maduro - Once a bus driver and union leader, he became the President of Venezuela, highlighting a dramatic rise from humble beginnings, though his leadership has been controversial.

You are not on this earth without a purpose. If you were born with a birth defect, it does not mean there is no hope; the Lord can use what you perceive as deficiencies for a greater purpose. Consider how the Lord can work through you, even amidst your weaknesses.

It is possible that you have faced mistreatment or disdain, leading to feelings of despair. In such times, it is important to put your trust in the Lord and to focus on Him. Remember that Jesus Himself was despised and treated unjustly; He often went unnoticed by those around Him. You are not alone in experiencing contempt; it has also happened to the Lord and His disciples. Therefore, stand firm in your faith, knowing that the Lord has the ability to uplift those who are marginalized or underestimated

You are here with a purpose, and it's important not to limit yourself based on perceived disabilities or the opinions of others. Regardless of any challenges you've faced or negativity directed at you, remember that each person's journey has meaning. Focus on your goals and aspirations, and seek guidance and strength from GOD.

By directing your attention toward positive outcomes and staying resilient, you have the potential to achieve great things. Embrace your journey and keep moving forward.

Chapter Eighteen

Let Us Not take pride in what fade Away

Proverbs 31:30 says, "Charm is deceptive, and beauty is fleeting; but a woman who fears the Lord is to be praised.

"Walk in the way of love, just as Christ loved us and gave himself up for us as a fragrant offering and sacrifice to God." — Ephesians 5:2

I remember one evening while watching TV, I came across something truly remarkable. I saw a woman named Mata Amritanandamayi, known simply as Amma. Her primary mission involves hugging people as she travels around the world. What struck me was her ability to connect with others without saying a word — just through the act of hugging. People lined up for hours, eager to receive her embrace. It was deeply moving to witness the joy on their faces, especially a nine-year-old boy who cried tears of happiness when she hugged him. The love she exuded seemed to emanate from her very being, offering comfort and healing to those around her.

Reflecting on her remarkable gift, I often find myself asking, "Why are we Christians sometimes unable to walk in genuine love?"

Personally, I enjoy hugging people out of a sincere desire to show love. Even when people are hesitant to greet me, I make the effort to hug and welcome them. Sadly, many of us harbor feelings of enmity, even while living under the roof of the church and claiming to be Christians. If we are to truly embody God's word, we must purge our hearts of hate and strive to walk in love.

I came across a quote that resonated with me: "Don't claim to be religious and a Christian when you are unkind and criticize or belittle others. Remember what God's word says about self-reflection and treating others with kindness. It's disheartening to see someone who points fingers and criticizes others while professing to be a churchgoer."

In a world that often feels divided, the call to walk in love serves as a powerful reminder of our shared humanity. It challenges us to embody the essence of Christ's love in our daily interactions.

Throughout my life, I have encountered many individuals, but what continually amazes me are those who claim to be Christians while harboring hatred and a critical spirit. These individuals often take on the role of faultfinders and judgmental observers, exaggerating the failures of others and making them public. Surprisingly, they are frequent attendees at church services, masking their true nature behind a façade of righteousness, aiming to appear virtuous in the eyes of others.

It is essential to recognize that the Word of God calls us to walk in love. Those of us who declare that we have been "born again" through faith in Jesus are expected to extend love and honor to our brothers and sisters. Merely attending church does not define a Christian; rather, it is our ability to emulate Jesus and treat others with love that truly reflects our faith. The manifestation of the fruits of the Spirit in our lives is a testament to our character.

As Nova L. Navonne Johns aptly stated, "A person's character is shown through their actions in life, not where they sit on Sunday."

We are called to inherit the character of Jesus, and it is evident that God grieves over how we sometimes treat one another. Instead of embodying love, we often find ourselves devouring, hating, and biting one another, rather than imitating the example set by Christ. In a world where everyone strives to be "better than others," we must remember that such attitudes are contrary to the spirit of love and unity that God desires for us.

Many come to church seeking refuge from the hate, deceit, and conflict prevalent in the world. They are in search of individuals who can show them genuine love and provide a sense of peace. It is our responsibility to extend love to those who find themselves in darkness and confusion. If we profess our love for Jesus yet fail to love our brothers and sisters, our lives become devoid of purpose.

The Word of the Lord says, "A new commandment I give to you, that you love one another: just as I have loved you, you also are to love one another. By this all people will know that you are my disciples, if you have love for one another" (John 13:34-35).

Jesus Christ has given us a commandment to love one another. As followers of Christ, it is essential that we observe this commandment and set an example for others. Our love and kindness should be distinguishing traits that identify us. When we walk in love, we contribute to peace within our neighborhoods and broader communities. May we seek the grace to live out this commandment.

Furthermore, Scripture reminds us, "And over all these virtues put on love, which binds them all together in perfect unity" (Colossians 3:14).

Chapter Nineteen

Walking In Love

"Walk in the way of love, just as Christ loved us and gave himself up for us as a fragrant offering and sacrifice to God." Ephesians 5:2.

I remember one evening while watching TV, I came across something truly remarkable. I saw a woman named Mata Amritanandamayi, known simply as Amma. Her primary mission involves hugging people as she travels around the world. What struck me was her ability to connect with others without saying a word — just through the act of hugging. People lined up for hours, eager to receive her embrace. It was deeply moving to witness the joy on their faces, especially a nine-year-old boy who cried tears of happiness when she hugged him. The love she exuded seemed to emanate from her very being, offering comfort and healing to those around her.

Reflecting on her remarkable gift, I often find myself asking, "Why are we Christians sometimes unable to walk in genuine love?"

Personally, I enjoy hugging people out of a sincere desire to show love. Even when people are hesitant to greet me, I make the effort to hug and welcome them. Sadly, many of us harbor feelings of enmity, even while living under the roof of the church and claiming to be Christians. If we are to truly embody God's word, we must purge our hearts of hate and strive to walk in love.

I came across a quote that resonated with me: "Don't claim to be religious and a Christian when you are unkind and criticize or belittle others. Remember what God's word says about self-reflection and treating others with kindness. It's disheartening to see someone who points fingers and criticizes others while professing to be a churchgoer."

In a world that often feels divided, the call to walk in love serves as a powerful reminder of our shared humanity. It challenges us to embody the essence of Christ's love in our daily interactions.

Throughout my life, I have encountered many individuals, but what continually amazes me are those who claim to be Christians while harboring hatred and a critical spirit. These individuals often take on the role of faultfinders and judgmental observers, exaggerating the failures of others and making them public. Surprisingly, they are frequent attendees at church services, masking their true nature behind a façade of righteousness, aiming to appear virtuous in the eyes of others.

It is essential to recognize that the Word of God calls us to walk in love. Those of us who declare that we have been "born again" through faith in Jesus are expected to extend love and honor to our brothers and sisters. Merely attending church does not define a Christian; rather, it is our ability to emulate Jesus and treat others with love that truly reflects our faith. The manifestation of the fruits of the Spirit in our lives is a testament to our character. As Nova L. Navonne Johns aptly stated, "A person's character is shown through their actions in life, not where they sit on Sunday."

We are called to inherit the character of Jesus, and it is evident that God grieves over how we sometimes treat one another. Instead of embodying love, we often find ourselves devouring, hating, and biting one another, rather than imitating the example set by Christ. In a world where everyone strives to be "better than others," we must remember that such attitudes are contrary to the spirit of love and unity that God desires for us.

Many come to church seeking refuge from the hate, deceit, and conflict prevalent in the world. They are in search of individuals who can show them genuine love and provide a sense of peace. It is our responsibility to extend love to those who find themselves in darkness and confusion. If we profess our love for Jesus yet fail to love our brothers and sisters, our lives become devoid of purpose.

The Word of the Lord says, "A new commandment I give to you, that you love one another: just as I have loved you, you also are to love one another. By this all people will know that you are my disciples, if you have love for one another" (John 13:34-35).

Jesus Christ has given us a commandment to love one another. As followers of Christ, it is essential that we observe this commandment and set an example for others. Our love and kindness should be distinguishing traits that identify us. When we walk in love, we contribute to peace within our neighborhoods and broader communities. May we seek the grace to live out this commandment.

Furthermore, Scripture reminds us, "And over all these virtues put on love, which binds them all together in perfect unity" (Colossians 3:14).

Chapter Twenty

A Life of Humility

"When pride comes, then comes disgrace, but with humility comes wisdom." Proverbs 11:2.

When pride comes, then comes disgrace, but with humility comes wisdom." — Proverbs 11:2.

Walking in humility may sometimes lead us to be belittled and despised. However, despite the negativity we may encounter, we will ultimately receive our reward from the Lord. It is important to continue walking in humility. One of my favorite sayings encapsulates this idea:

"Humility is not thinking less of yourself; it is thinking of yourself less." — C.S. Lewis

"It was pride that changed angels into devils; it is humility that makes us as angels." — Augustine of Hippo.

My mother has taught me many valuable lessons. She is educated and beautiful, an intelligent, God-fearing, and prayerful woman. Each day, she dedicates hours to prayer before going to work and upon returning home. God is always her priority.

She supports others generously with her time, money, and love. Unfortunately, I have seen some people misunderstand her humility and love, mistaking them for ignorance.

This often saddens me, but she consistently maintains a positive attitude toward others. She often tells me, "Be kind all the time; do what is expected of you; if they are evil, it is their business." Her mind is bright, and she has never shied away from love and kindness. Although she is not well-known by many, the Lord is aware of her kindness, love, and generosity.

I have learned a lot from my mother, one of the most important lessons being to expect nothing from anyone. She was beautiful, knowledgeable, and wealthy; she could have easily taken pride in these attributes. Instead, she held onto Jesus Christ tightly, understanding that all these things are temporary and will ultimately perish. What benefits us most is not glorifying our knowledge, beauty, or wealth, but glorifying our God. No one who has held onto Jesus has ever been put to shame.

My father, on the other hand, did not believe in Christ and was not born again. Although he was highly educated, he did not regularly attend church. Nevertheless, he has always supported others with humility and possesses a very humble spirit. He is loving and treats all people equally, never taking pride in his knowledge or skills. His ability to live harmoniously with everyone is remarkable. I often see the Lord's character reflected in him. What he has imparted to us, his children, are values such as treating all people equally, humility, love, goodness, and kindness. Particularly, we have learned to love others from his example. I encourage you to pass these values on to your children.

As Orison Swett Marden wisely said, "The man who practices unselfishness, who is genuinely interested in the welfare of others, who feels it a privilege to have the power to do a fellow creature a kindness—even though polished manners and a gracious presence may be absent—will be an elevating influence wherever he goes."

Let us not become conceited, showing contempt for one another or making claims such as, "My ethnicity is better than yours," "I am superior," "I am educated," or "I am beautiful."

God commands us to be humble, and in the same breath, He promises to grant us power, position, and glory.

In 1 Peter 5:5-6, the call to humility is clear: younger individuals are encouraged to submit to their elders, and everyone is urged to be humble and supportive of one another. The passage emphasizes that God resists the proud but bestows grace on those who are humble, highlighting the importance of humility in our relationship with God and others.

Ephesians 4:1-2 further reinforces this idea, urging believers to embody humility and gentleness, to be patient, and to bear with one another in love. This suggests that humility is foundational not only in our spiritual lives but also in our interactions within the community.

If we desire trustworthy leaders, friendly neighbors, and obedient children, humility is essential. According to Richard Foster in The Worthy Walk of Humility, genuine humility must be reflected in our everyday interactions, whether with colleagues, family, or service staff.

In Philippians 2:3-4, the scripture instructs believers to act without selfish ambition and to prioritize the interests of others, again pointing to the significance of humility in fostering healthy relationships. Similarly, Colossians 3:12 encourages individuals to adorn themselves with qualities like compassion and kindness, which are rooted in a humble spirit.

While some may mock or criticize humility, it is important to remain steadfast in this virtue. Ultimately, walking in humility is not only a directive from scripture but also a means to honor God in our lives.

From my mother, father, brothers and a beloved sister in the Lord who is no longer with me, I have learned the importance of respecting and loving others.

I once knew a couple whom I admired greatly. They were both well-educated and financially secure, exemplifying an ideal partnership. When they invited people to their home for meals, they did not focus on well-known individuals or those who might bring gifts. Instead, they often welcomed those who were unknown, ostracized, neglected, or marginalized. Throughout their lives, they embodied humility, patience, love, compassion, and kindness.

The experience I have shared highlights the profound impact of humility, love, and respect in our relationships with others. The couple I mentioned exemplifies the value of reaching out to those who are often overlooked, demonstrating that true worth is found not in status or material possessions, but in compassion and kindness. Their practice of inviting those who are marginalized reflects a deep understanding of the importance of inclusivity and belonging.

There was another sister who, while she was still alive, fell ill and was admitted to the hospital. A large number of people came to visit her, and due to the influx of visitors, security guards monitored the entrance to prevent overcrowding. The reason for the large turnout was her humility; she consistently fed, offered drinks to, visited, befriended, and clothed those in need. Her character reflected the values she held dear, as she radiated humility, patience, and love wherever she went. Because she honored the Lord, she received honor in return. She was well-loved by all, and her home was a source of blessings; she experienced abundance in her life.

The sister in the hospital illustrates how humility and generosity can create a strong community bond. Her willingness to care for others, provide for their needs, and build genuine relationships fostered a network of love and support that drew many to her during a time of need. This serves as a reminder that our actions and attitudes can have a significant influence on those around us, often leading to a legacy of kindness and respect.

My parents exhibited similar qualities. This poses a question for reflection: What values and behaviors are we passing on to our children, neighbors, colleagues, and our community?

Ultimately, the values we embody—whether humility, respect, love, or compassion—become the foundation for how we interact with others and how we are remembered. They serve as powerful lessons that, when passed on, can significantly impact future generations and contribute to a more caring and supportive community.

May we strive to follow the example of humility set by Jesus, recognizing that the Lord's watchful presence is upon us. We are called to walk in humility, as highlighted in Scripture: "He does not take His eyes off the righteous; He enthrones them with kings and exalts them forever" (Job 36:7). This assurance reminds us that when we embody humility and kindness, we align ourselves with God's expectations, and in return, we find His support. The Word of God encourages us to "pursue righteousness; strive to do what is good."

It is true that finding individuals who demonstrate kindness and maintain a good conscience can be challenging. We may face disdain from others, but such reactions should not deter us. As Scripture states, "We are fools for Christ, but you are so wise in Christ! We are weak, but you are strong! You are honored; we are dishonored! To this very hour we go hungry and thirsty; we are in rags, we are brutally treated, we are homeless. We work hard with our own hands. When we are cursed, we bless; when we are

persecuted, we endure; when we are slandered, we respond kindly. We have become the scum of the earth, the garbage of the world—right up to this moment"
(1 Corinthians 4:10-13).

Practicing daily acts of kindness is a meaningful way to reflect humility in interactions with others. Simple gestures, such as offering a compliment, listening attentively, or helping someone with a task, can make a significant impact on those around us. These actions demonstrate a willingness to prioritize the needs and feelings of others, fostering a spirit of connection and understanding.

Engaging in acts of kindness can be as straightforward as holding the door open for someone, expressing gratitude, or offering emotional support to a friend. By consistently being mindful of how we treat others, we not only promote positivity in our immediate environment but also cultivate a culture of kindness and respect.

Additionally, practicing humility in our interactions can help us approach others with an open mind and heart, allowing for deeper connections and more meaningful relationships. By acknowledging our shared humanity, we contribute to a more compassionate community.

Chapter Twenty One

Sharing with others what has been done for us

I cannot refrain from speaking about what I have seen, heard, and experienced, just like the apostles who said, "We cannot help speaking about what we have seen and heard." (Acts 4:20)

"My Lord Jesus Christ, whom I love and honor, You chose me without my choosing You; You loved me without my loving You. You showed me Your love by being crucified on a cross and delivered me from many challenges. My dear Lord, how can I repay Your favor? I glorify Your name by sharing with others what You have done for me and exalting You. I thank You because You are my joy, protector, friend, advocate, and healer. You have borne with me, and You will never grow weary of me.

I lift up Your name with the saints who are devoted to glorifying You. I will speak of Your name and Your fame forever. I will proclaim Your name alongside the saints for all eternity; I praise You, I exalt You, and I glorify You forever.

I will glorify Your name not because of what You have given me or done for me, but because You are worthy. I am grateful for the opportunity You have given me to worship and serve You.

Help me to communicate the love, patience, and kindness that fill my innermost being. Amen!"

Speak of the Lord Jesus Christ continually; let His presence be evident in your life. I am certain there are countless things He has done for us. In remembering His deeds, let each of us exalt Christ. Do not despair; live each day as if it were your last on earth. Express your appreciation for every good thing God has done for you.

Do not hesitate to speak about who the Lord Jesus Christ is whenever an opportunity arises. Exalt His holy name tirelessly. The biblical story of the Samaritan woman serves as a perfect example. Her account is found in John 4:6-34. In the days of His earthly ministry, the Lord Jesus Christ traveled to Sychar, a town in Samaria. He was weary from His journey and sat down by Jacob's well, a location where the people of Samaria came to draw water. Around noon, a Samaritan woman arrived to fetch water, and Jesus asked her for a drink. Taken aback, she responded, "You are a Jew, and I am a Samaritan woman. How can you ask me for a drink?" This was because, during that time, Jews and

Samaritans generally did not associate with one another and often held contempt for each other.

The woman only perceived Jesus as a Jew, and her spiritual eyes had yet to be opened. However, the Lord replied, "If you knew who it is that asks you for a drink, you would have asked Him, and He would have given you living water." Despite His words, she struggled to grasp their meaning.

When Jesus spoke to the Samaritan woman about spiritual matters, she focused on earthly concerns. When He mentioned, "I will give you living water," she responded, "The well is deep; how can you get this living water?" She further questioned, "Are you greater than our father Jacob, who gave us this well?"

After some discussion, the Lord Jesus revealed something profound about her life—something she sought after but could not attain. She was a woman who had tried many paths in search of joy, yet none had fulfilled her. Knowing her deep longing for eternal joy, peace, and salvation, Jesus said to her, "Go, call your husband and come back."

She replied, "I have no husband." Jesus responded, "You have had five husbands, and the one you now have is not your husband." At this revelation, she ceased her argument and acknowledged Him, saying, "You are a prophet." She continued, "I know that the Messiah called Christ is coming; when He comes, He will explain everything to us." Jesus then declared, "I, the one speaking to you, am He."

Jesus continued, "Everyone who drinks of this water will be thirsty again, but whoever drinks of the water that I will give him will never be thirsty again. The water that I will give him will become in him a spring of water welling up to eternal life."

Following her conversation with Jesus, the Samaritan woman accepted the "living water" He offered. She felt a deep affection for Him after He revealed truths about her life without judgment. His candid yet loving approach astonished her, and she couldn't contain her gratitude for His kindness. Leaving her water jar behind, she hurried back to her town to share her experience with others.

Upon her arrival, she recounted what Jesus had done for her, urging the townspeople, "Come and see the Lord Jesus Christ." She spoke about Him to everyone she encountered. Many Samaritans came to believe in Him because of her testimony. As a result of her influence, numerous women and men in the town embraced faith in Jesus. They expressed their desire for Him to stay with them, and the compassion and mercy of Jesus resonated deeply within them.

Eventually, the townspeople acknowledged her impact, stating, "We no longer believe just because of your word; we ourselves have seen the Lord Jesus Christ; we have met Him in person." This affirmation marked a significant moment of communal faith in the area.

The people of Samaria expressed their gratitude to the woman by acknowledging that their belief was no longer solely based on her testimony but on their personal experiences with Jesus. They proclaimed their recognition of Him as the Christ and the Savior of the world. This highlights an important aspect of faith—personal encounters with the divine often deepen understanding and belief.

Reflecting on the question of why individuals today may struggle to share their faith can be a valuable exercise. Various factors might contribute to this, including societal norms, fear of rejection, or a lack of confidence in articulating their beliefs. It's crucial for believers to consider how their own experiences with Jesus could motivate them to share their faith with others, especially those who may be in spiritual darkness.

The example set by the disciples illustrates the importance of consistently proclaiming faith, regardless of the circumstances. Their dedication to openly discussing and promoting Jesus serves as a reminder that sharing one's beliefs can be an integral part of being a follower of Christ. Engaging with others about faith can happen in many contexts, and doing so can encourage and inspire those around us.

As a woman who struggles to articulate my thoughts verbally, I find my heart filled with love for those around me. I strive to live in harmony with others and approach each person with respect and kindness. Many who get to know me often ask, "Why are you so full of joy?" I take these opportunities to share about my Lord and Savior, Jesus Christ. I make it a point not to judge or condemn anyone; instead, I aim to present myself with humility and grace. Those drawn to me are often those in need of love and acceptance, and I believe that living out virtues like love, patience, kindness, and humility allows the light of Jesus to shine through me.

When we embody these qualities, people may naturally gravitate toward us and inquire about the source of our joy and peace. It's important to remember that we don't have to be in traditional public settings to share our faith. Our lifestyles can enact change and inspire others through their beauty and authenticity.

One individual once expressed their struggle with sharing their testimony about Jesus, stating that in their environment, people often respond with skepticism, asking, "What can I help you with?" They shared that, despite having a message of hope, those in their life perceive them as a sad or pessimistic person, which makes it challenging to communicate their faith.

It's true that if our conversations revolve primarily around complaints and challenges, others may be less receptive to hearing about the Lord. To effectively witness, it's essential for us to be approachable and inviting. Those around us are always observing our attitudes and behaviors, often drawing conclusions about our character long before we engage in deeper dialogue.

Reflecting on my past, I remember living in a small apartment where I made it a habit to greet my neighbors and engage with those I encountered, even in an elevator. One day, while I was cooking, I accidentally burned the food.

As I opened the door to let the odor dissipate, I carried on with my day, washing dishes that had piled up in the sink.

At that moment, something happened that stays with me to this day.

A Muslim woman, wearing a covering on her face, brought her lifeless 8-month-old child into my apartment, placing the child on the sink. Distressed and tearful, she pleaded with me, "My child has died; his eyes are closed; he is not breathing; I beg you, please help me; do something for me." In shock, I found myself praying, "You child, rise up in the name of the Lord Jesus Christ," while the woman continued to cry out for help. Neighbors quickly gathered in my apartment and began calling 911. I hadn't thought to call for help myself; my immediate instinct was to pray.

As I continued to invoke the name of Jesus Christ, remarkably, the child began to breathe and opened his eyes. The mother, visibly relieved, started thanking me in both English and Arabic as Emergency Medical Services (EMS) arrived to assist her and the baby.

After the incident, she mentioned that she had two other children, prompting me to check on them at her home. Questions swirled in my mind: "Why didn't she call 911 first? Why did she come to my apartment?" I resolved to ask her once she returned.
When I inquired, she explained, "When I saw my baby in that state, I panicked. In that emotional turmoil, Allah led

me to your home; that's why I brought him here." She then asked, "What is it that you said that saved my child?" I told her, "I called upon the name of Jesus, the name above all names." This conversation led to discussions about faith, and from that day, we began to pray together privately.

This experience served as a powerful reminder of the connections we can form in moments of deep distress and the ways in which faith can intersect in our lives.

I shared this story to illustrate how people observe our way of life. The Lord provided me with the opportunity to share my faith with a woman I encountered. As I mentioned, we can testify about the Lord in various ways.

David writes, "My mouth will tell of your righteous deeds, of your saving acts all day long—though I know not how to relate them all. I will come and proclaim your mighty acts, Sovereign Lord; I will proclaim your righteous deeds, yours alone. Since my youth, God, you have taught me, and to this day I declare your marvelous deeds. Even when I am old and gray, do not forsake me, my God, till I declare your power to the next generation, your mighty acts to all who are to come" (Psalms 71:15-18).

In this passage, David expresses his desire to not be forsaken in old age until he can share what God has done for him with future generations. Each of us needs to embrace David's prayer.

"Lord, you know that my lips will not be silent. I will not keep your kindness to myself; I will speak about your love and faithfulness. I will not hide your love and truth from others. Do not withhold your mercy from me. May your love watch over all who seek your truth. Amen."

The testimonies I share about how God has worked in my life have provided encouragement and comfort to those facing similar situations.

My experiences through many trying situations have shown me that God is working more actively within me each day.

I have realized that in doing so, He is multiplying the fruits of the Spirit within me, making me more like Him and transforming my life. He is instilling in me love, joy, peace, patience, kindness, and self-control. I will never cease to testify about my Lord Jesus Christ until I finish my race and draw my last breath. My desire to share fully what the Lord has done for me is strong. May God help each of us to speak about Him through our songs and platforms, and in every way available to us.

"Your testimony is like a key to a prison that unlocks a prisoner. God uses the hands and feet of men." — Charles Spurgeon.

I encourage you to share the story of God freely and clearly at all times. When we speak about what God has done in our lives, we remember His kindness and goodness. Recalling His past deeds fills us with greater faith and confidence in the present. When God led the Israelites out of Egypt, their remembrance of His actions bolstered their courage to continue their journey to the Promised Land. Similarly, the disciples of Jesus recalled His teachings and shared them with others. Understanding their responsibility to spread Jesus' message empowered them to tell many about the way of the Lord through their own experiences.

1 Peter 3:15-16 emphasizes the importance of recognizing Christ as the Lord of one's life and the need to be prepared to explain one's hope in Him to others. It encourages believers to respond with gentleness and respect, maintaining a clear conscience in their interactions.

The passage underscores the idea that suffering for doing good is preferable to suffering for wrongdoing, suggesting that one's actions and demeanor can have a positive impact on how others perceive their faith. This teaching invites reflection on how to embody Christ's values in everyday situations and engage in meaningful conversations about one's beliefs.

Chapter Twenty Two

Approachable Spirit

As believers, our everyday actions and demeanor should serve as an example to others. Our lives should naturally attract those around us.

One of my earnest prayers to the Lord is for the grace to cultivate a spirit and personality that draws people in. Some may argue, "This is an innate quality; if I wasn't born with it, I can't develop that kind of approachable spirit." However, I believe this is a trait we can learn and embrace.

Even negative traits can be learned; for instance, a person engaged in wrongdoing often speaks about their actions as if they were commendable. By fostering an approachable personality, we can connect with and captivate others more easily.

Let me share a story from my childhood. I knew a girl named Belu who had a deep love for the Lord. However, she also held a serious and often judgmental demeanor. She would frequently admonish me, saying, "What do you need with all these worldly friends? The Word of God teaches that light cannot associate with darkness. Wongel, I worry that God's wrath may fall upon you."

In reflecting on her perspective, I learned that we must balance our faith with an approachable spirit. It's important to welcome others with love and understanding rather than judgment. This openness can lead to meaningful connections and opportunities for sharing our beliefs.

I was 13 years old at the time, while Belu was 18. I admired her greatly; everything she did fascinated me, especially her prayer life. The Spirit of the Lord worked powerfully through her. At such a young age, she would frequently get into a taxi or stand by the roadside to preach, boldly declaring, "Jesus is Lord." Often, she returned home with injuries from stones thrown at her. I felt sympathy for her, but despite the persecution and suffering she faced, she never wavered in her commitment to testify about the Lord. She would often remind me, "We are destined to be persecuted for His name's sake," reflecting her deep love for Jesus Christ.

However, she faced a challenge: she found it difficult to make friends, as many people were intimidated by her fervor. Yet, she remained unconcerned about this. When I asked her, "Why do people not approach you?" she would reply, "When does Satan approach a person who loves the

Lord?" Since I wasn't allowed to go outside much, I eagerly awaited her return home, excited to hear about the people she had spoken to about Jesus and the experiences she had encountered in her ministry.

Although I wasn't allowed to go outside, I had many friends. There was an evangelist named Tesfaye who would visit our home to share the word of God and pray for us. He always prayed for the children I knew, and as a result, many of them came to accept the Lord. Belu once asked me, "Where do you find all these children?" To be honest, I wasn't quite sure. Whenever a child happened to come by, I would quickly make a connection with them, and the next day, they would return with two more friends. My circle of friends kept growing, as I was approachable and easy to connect with. All the children I befriended eventually believed in the Lord and began serving Him.

In contrast, Belu's approach to sharing her faith was different. She would often speak harshly about others' beliefs, warning them, "You will perish," which led to frustration and often resulted in people throwing stones at her. Her challenge seemed to be a lack of wisdom in how she approached others and shared the Gospel in a more engaging way.

Although I was not allowed to go outside, I had many friends. There was an evangelist named Tesfaye who would visit our house to share the word of God and pray with us. He never left without praying for the young people I knew.

Following his prayers, many of them accepted the Lord. Belu once asked me, "Where do you find all these friends?" To be honest, I wasn't quite sure where they came from. Whenever someone—young, old, or middle-aged—came to our house by chance, I would quickly make a connection with them, and the next day, they would often return with two more friends. My circle of friends kept expanding, as I had an approachable personality. All the individuals I mentioned eventually came to believe in the Lord and are now serving Him.

In contrast, Belu's approach to sharing her faith was different. She often warned others by saying, "You will perish," and criticized their beliefs, which caused frustration and led people to throw stones at her. Her challenge seemed to stem from a lack of wisdom in how to approach others and share the Gospel in a more engaging way.

When we approach people in a manner that is acceptable to them, they often express their desire to worship the God we worship without us having to prompt them. Change cannot be enforced through force or intimidation. I strive to be friends with everyone, regardless of their religion, ethnicity, or socioeconomic status. As a result, I am respected by those around me, and I genuinely respect them in return. When the time is right, they may ask me, "Can we go to church with you?" and I gladly respond, "Of course." If they show interest and say, "Introduce us to your Lord.

Let us try your Lord Jesus Christ," I respond positively, "Yes." I have never judged them or belittled their beliefs. How can we effectively engage people if we do not maintain an approachable spirit?

The sister I mentioned earlier has undergone a transformation; she has changed her attitude and recognized that stubbornness and overly serious behavior are not helpful. As a result, she has also gained many friends.

A brother once expressed to me his strong desire to serve the Lord, stating, "I want to serve the Lord so much, but nobody approaches me, even when I try to reach out. People tend to avoid me because I come across as serious. How can I serve the Lord or testify about Him? I've attempted to preach in various public places, like trains and buses, but nothing seemed to work. If I don't have a platform, people are reluctant to engage with me."

I replied, "You don't necessarily need to go to public places or have a formal platform. People can be influenced by the fruits of the Spirit that are evident in your life. It's important to approach others with love, to lighten up a bit, and to smile more. Building relationships is a gradual process, and by being non-judgmental, there's no reason why people would not want to connect with you." However, when we met again after some time, it became clear from our conversation that he had not experienced any significant changes in his situation.

One of the reasons we may not see new individuals joining the church is that they often do not feel welcomed into the fellowship of believers. This can be due to a lack of outreach to those outside the church who have not yet experienced the light of the gospel. It is important for us to be present for those in need, offering our testimony about the love of Christ through both words and actions.

Often, our focus remains on our own group, leaving little concern for those outside, even as we witness their struggles. This is not in alignment with the character of Jesus. We need to move beyond this mindset and extend our support to those who are hurting or facing adversity. Only then can we truly glorify Jesus. It is my ongoing prayer that we can reach beyond ourselves to assist and uplift others.

When we approach people with love and embody the essence of the Lord Jesus Christ, we can inspire curiosity and interest. Others may find themselves drawn to our joy and peace, prompting questions such as, "What is your secret to happiness?" or "How do you maintain such kindness and humility?" It is through these interactions that we can open the door to meaningful conversations about salvation and faith.

In Acts 13:46-52, we read, "The disciples were filled with joy and with the Holy Spirit." May God bless us with this kind of abundant life. When our hearts are filled with love, God fills them with joy. However, when our hearts are filled with craftiness and wickedness, joy has no place in our lives, leaving us riddled with puzzles. When our lives are filled with confusion, we lack the strength to be examples to others. Some individuals effortlessly make friends and connect with many because they possess a welcoming attitude, which makes them well-liked by others.

At one point, a Habesha girl was employed at the company where I worked. Without exaggeration, she was truly beautiful. My boss approached me and said, "I've hired a girl who looks like you; I think you may be from the same country. I'll introduce you to her tomorrow, and if you like her, I can send her to your department." At the time, I was working in customer service and eagerly anticipated meeting this girl. The next day, I went to her department and greeted her in Amharic, saying, "How are you?" She replied in Amharic, "Fine," and then switched to English, saying, "I cannot speak Amharic; I can only speak English. I am Eritrean, not Ethiopian." I was taken aback and thought to myself, "What an attitude." I simply responded, "Nice to meet you," and returned to my desk.

A few days later, my boss approached my desk and asked, "How is she?" I replied, "I would prefer it if you did not send her to my section." He inquired, "Why?" and I explained, "I did not find her attitude appealing." He responded, "Really?" I confirmed my feelings and he suggested, "Let's observe her for three months, and if she is unfit, I will let her go." I agreed, saying, "That sounds like a good idea."

I generally do not appreciate prideful behavior, which my colleagues were aware of. When there were no customers, they would often come to my desk to talk, laugh, and spend time together. As the girl observed this interaction, she began to notice the closeness among my colleagues and me. Gradually, she started to come to my section more frequently. However, I maintained my distance, especially since she had expressed that she did not want to form close relationships with anyone.

Some time later, she approached me and asked, "Can you speak Amharic or Tigrinya?" I replied, "I cannot." She then said, "I'm sorry for my attitude" in English. In response, I hugged her, thinking to myself, "This is what makes her pleasant." However, when I tried to let go, she held on. I asked her, "Is everything alright?" She then spoke to me in Amharic, saying, "I have many things to tell you."

I agreed and took her out for coffee during our break. I asked her, "Why did you initially say you couldn't speak Amharic?" She explained, "I did that deliberately. My parents taught me not to get close to Habesha people because they had been hurt by many of them. My father speaks Amharic; he is the one who taught it to me."

She then confided in me, tearfully sharing her secret. In that moment, I understood the source of her previously difficult behavior and the reasons behind her attitude. From that day onward, we became close friends. I made it a point to include her in our section at work, and my boss often smiled whenever he saw us together. After eight months of working together, she moved to Vancouver.

At first, this girl didn't want to get close to me, but her perspective changed when she observed the connections I had with others and the affection they showed me. It's true that people often take time to evaluate others before forming relationships. When you treat everyone with kindness and warmth, they are more likely to be drawn to you. Even if they might not have feelings for you initially, your loving treatment toward others can encourage them to approach you. While you may not be expected to befriend everyone, it is important to embody a character that attracts people. The principle from the Word reminds us, "If possible, as far as it depends on you, live peaceably with everyone." Therefore, let us strive to walk in love and peace with those around us.

Years ago, I had a neighbor who was a Mormon. She and her friends frequently knocked on my door, asking me to join them. Initially, I welcomed them whenever they came by. However, as our discussions continued, I found their messages increasingly unappealing. Eventually, I chose not to open the door to them anymore and started avoiding interactions. One day, my neighbor called out, "Wongel, open the door; I know you're in there." Feeling annoyed, I reluctantly opened the door. She then asked, "Why are you annoyed? Are you alright?"

I replied to her, "I don't judge people; I prefer to live a life filled with love. However, you frequently come here asking me to convert to your religion, which annoys me and makes me resistant to your beliefs. I have one Lord, Jesus Christ, whom I love, honor, and worship. He is my source of joy and beauty. I worship and bow down to no one else but Him; He alone is my God. While you've shared your beliefs about your religion, now I want to share about my Lord Jesus Christ."

She responded with an "Okay," and I continued to explain who Jesus is to me.

After I spoke, she remarked, "We know Jesus, but he's not quite as you describe him. It's clear that you have a deep fellowship with Him, and that's quite inspiring. I didn't realize you had such a profound connection with the Lord and that your focus is so clearly on Him."

I continued, "He is the peace-giver, helper, friend..." Before I could finish, she began to tear up. She shared with me, "What I mainly lack is peace. I grew up in a dysfunctional family and didn't receive love from my family. As a result, I sought validation in relationships, thinking that men who complimented me truly cared for me. This led to a cycle of dissatisfaction, and I turned to alcohol as an escape. I eventually met someone involved in Mormonism, who introduced me to the faith. Yet, I still couldn't find the peace I was looking for. When I confided in fellow Mormons about my struggles, they told me it was Satan preventing my peace and suggested I share my faith door-to-door. So, I began doing that, but I still felt lost. I wondered, 'How can I find peace?

'When you shared about Jesus, something shifted within me; I felt like a weight had been lifted. That's why I'm crying—I sensed the presence of Jesus."

I prayed in tongues and told her, "The peace Jesus gives is inexhaustible and eternal. Receive Him and drink from this unfailing source; you'll be set free from whatever binds you. Remember Matthew 11:28: 'Come to me, all you who are weary and burdened, and I will give you rest.'" After we prayed, she left. From that point onward, she didn't come by to discuss her religion but instead visited to share meals and enjoy time together.

She informed her Mormon friends not to visit my house. She embraced belief in Jesus and began attending a church where the true Lord Jesus Christ is worshipped. The reason I share these stories is to emphasize the importance of having an approachable spirit and personality.

We cannot effectively lead others to the Lord by despising or judging them. If I hadn't reached out to the individuals I mentioned earlier, they may not have given me the opportunity to discuss my faith with them. We are called to be light and salt in a world that is in need.

The motivation for sharing these experiences is to highlight the importance of maintaining an open and inviting demeanor. An approachable attitude can foster meaningful connections and discussions, particularly in matters of faith. It emphasizes the idea that kindness and understanding can create opportunities for dialogue and understanding, allowing individuals to explore different perspectives more freely.

Fostering a warm and approachable attitude is crucial for building strong interpersonal connections. Such an attitude creates a welcoming environment, making others feel valued and respected. This can lead to open communication and the sharing of ideas, which is especially important in discussions involving personal beliefs or experiences. When individuals feel comfortable approaching one another, it encourages dialogue, understanding, and collaboration, ultimately strengthening relationships and fostering a sense of community. An approachable demeanor can help bridge differences and facilitate constructive conversations across diverse perspectives.

Chapter Twenty Three

How to Raise Our Children?

Raising children entails significant responsibilities. As parents, we hold the primary role in their upbringing, prompting the essential question: How should we guide our children?

"Children are a heritage from the Lord, offspring a reward from him." - Psalms 127:3

important topic of raising children, emphasizing the responsibilities that come with parenthood. It draws on the idea that children are considered blessings, highlighting the significance of approaching child-rearing with care and thoughtfulness.

The chapter explores several key points:

1. Child-Centered Decisions: Parents are urged to make decisions that prioritize the well-being and needs of their children. This includes not only material provisions such as education, food, and clothing but also emotional support and understanding.

2. Responsibility: The text underscores that bringing children into the world comes with a commitment to raise them properly. Parents are encouraged to reflect on their choices and how these choices impact their children's lives. 3. Recognizing Feelings: It is noted that children have their own feelings and emotions that deserve acknowledgment. The chapter critiques the notion that providing for children's basic needs is sufficient, stressing the importance of listening to children and valuing their perspectives.

4. Community Perspective: The text recognizes the sacrifices parents make and highlights cultural aspects of parenting, suggesting that child-rearing practices often stem from community values.

Overall, the chapter advocates for a holistic approach to raising children, where emotional and psychological needs are considered alongside physical care, encouraging parents to foster an environment of love, support, and mutual respect.

Prioritizing Child-Centered Decisions

Children are a precious gift, and it is our duty to nurture this gift responsibly. We bring them into the world without their consent, thereby assuming full responsibility for their well-being.

Raising children often requires us to make sacrifices, prioritizing their needs over our own. As parents, we must be mindful of every choice we make, ensuring that it considers their best interests. Merely providing for their physical needs, such as education, food, and clothing, is not enough; we must also attend to their emotional well-being. Children, full of innocence and joy, deserve our unwavering support and attention.

I admire the sacrifices made by parents in our community, who strive to fulfill their children's desires while also instilling discipline. However, it is crucial to recognize that children have feelings too. Often, we overlook their emotional needs, operating under the belief that meeting their basic needs suffices for their obedience and respect. Listening to children and valuing their thoughts and emotions should be integral to parenting.

Child-Centered Decisions

Making child-centered decisions is a fundamental aspect of effective parenting. This approach emphasizes prioritizing the needs and well-being of children in all facets of their upbringing. It acknowledges that children rely on adults not only for their physical necessities but also for their emotional and psychological development.

In practice, being child-centered entails that parents consider their children's interests, feelings, and perspectives when making decisions. This includes choices related to education, healthcare, extracurricular activities, and daily routines. Such decisions should aim to support a child's overall development and happiness.

Engaging children in discussions about matters that impact them is essential, as it can help them feel valued and heard. Actively listening to their opinions and emotions can lead to healthier family dynamics and foster better understanding between parents and children.

Additionally, child-centered decisions often involve setting boundaries and expectations while also allowing for appropriate autonomy and independence based on the child's age and maturity level. Striking this balance promotes responsibility and helps children develop their decision-making skills.

Ultimately, prioritizing child-centered decisions contributes to a nurturing environment that fosters a child's growth and development, leading to stronger and healthier parent-child relationships.

It's important to recognize that children are affected by major family decisions, such as moving to a new country, changing schools, or switching churches. Often, parents may not consider the implications these changes have on their children's emotional well-being and sense of stability.

Parents might view such decisions as straightforward and may believe that involving children in discussions is unnecessary or time-consuming. However, it can be beneficial for parents to engage their children in conversations about significant changes that could impact their lives.

For instance, moving from one church to another might seem like a minor decision to parents, but for children, it can introduce feelings of confusion and loss, particularly if they have established friendships and a sense of belonging within their current church community.

Communicating openly about the reasons behind changes can help children understand the situation better and feel included in the decision-making process. Parents can discuss their preferences while also considering what is best for the children. For example, rather than simply transferring to a church that the parents prefer, they could evaluate together the benefits of remaining in a community where their children feel comfortable and supported.

Ultimately, parents bear the responsibility of ensuring that their children's needs are met, and sometimes this may mean making sacrifices for the sake of their children's emotional and social development. Engaging in these discussions not only helps children feel valued but also fosters a closer family bond grounded in mutual respect and understanding.

It's essential to recognize the significance of involving children in discussions about major decisions that may affect their lives. Decisions such as moving to another country, changing schools, or switching churches can have a considerable impact on a child's sense of stability and emotional well-being.

For instance, when parents are dissatisfied with their current church, they might opt to transition to a new one without consulting their children. While this decision may seem straightforward to adults, it can create confusion and insecurity for children who have formed attachments and friendships in their current environment.

Communicating the reasons behind such changes is vital. Parents should take the time to explain why they feel a change is necessary and how it aligns with the family's values and needs. It's important to consider the children's perspectives and feelings during these discussions, as this can help foster understanding and acceptance of the decisions being made.

Furthermore, when evaluating options like a new church, parents may benefit from prioritizing the needs and preferences of their children. Discussing the question, "Which church will be more beneficial for our children?" can help parents make informed choices that take into account their children's emotional attachments and social circles. Sometimes, this requires parents to make sacrifices for the well-being of their children, ensuring that their choices support a nurturing environment as children grow. Ultimately, being mindful of children's feelings and including them in these conversations reflects a commitment to child-centered decision-making, which can enhance family dynamics and provide children with a sense of security in times of change.

Your reflections on the impact of parental decisions regarding religious practices and community involvement on children are thought-provoking. Moving children between different church environments can indeed create confusion and emotional distress for some, as consistency and stability often contribute to a child's sense of security and identity.

It's important to recognize that children, as individuals with their own feelings and perspectives, should ideally be supported in ways that foster their joy and emotional well-being. When parents make decisions without considering the child's preferences, it can lead to feelings of disconnection or frustration.

Your reference to Genesis 33:4-5 highlights an important biblical perspective on children as gifts from God, emphasizing the responsibility parents have in nurturing and caring for them. This perspective underlines the need for thoughtful consideration in how decisions impact their development and happiness.

Ultimately, fostering an environment where children feel valued and heard can contribute positively to their emotional and psychological development. Encouraging open communication between parents and children can be beneficial in ensuring that children feel supported in their spiritual and personal journeys.

Causing children to wander from one church to another can have adverse effects on their minds. The more parents engage in this practice, the more confused the children may become. This can lead to instability in their emotional and psychological development, which should not be the case, and it is not our right to impose such turmoil on them. Often, children have no choice but to attend places they do not wish to go because their parents make the decisions. Over time, their joy can decline, and they may begin to display new, concerning behaviors.

I have spoken with many children and parents, and it saddens me to see children stripped of their joy at such a tender age. Children are not mere objects; they are gifts from God.

Genesis 33:4-5 states, "But Esau ran to meet Jacob and embraced him; he threw his arms around his neck and kissed him. And they wept. Then Esau looked up and saw the women and children. 'Who are these with you?' he asked. Jacob answered, 'They are the children God has graciously given your servant.'" When Esau saw the women and Jacob's children, he inquired about their identities.

Jacob responded, "They are the children God has graciously given your servant." Who gave them? It is God. He has entrusted us with these precious children as gifts. Praise be to His name! Therefore, we must take care of God's gifts.

I recall a particular instance involving a 9-year-old girl who exhibited significant changes in her behavior. She became depressed, and her mother grew increasingly worried about her well-being. The mother asked me to speak with her daughter, and during our conversation, the girl expressed, "My parents are only concerned about their own preferences. Since I was born, we've been moving from one church to another. This is how I have grown up. Whenever I make a friend in one church and start to feel comfortable, we leave and move to another. My brother and I have suffered a lot because of this. I do not like the church we are attending now; I go there only because my parents like it. I enjoyed the previous church, but my parents make decisions without discussing them with us. When we try to talk to them, they often say, 'You have to listen to us; you must abide by what we say.' We feel powerless. If we don't comply, they become angry, and this frightens us. I cannot connect with friends from the other church because my parents do not attend there. As a result, I feel depressed and constrained to do things I do not want to do just to make my parents happy; my brother feels the same way. If we refuse to go to church, they become very upset with us. We feel lost and unhappy due to the decisions they have made regarding our lives, which has led us to resent church."

I shared her feelings with her parents, and to their credit, they responded positively, stating, "From now on, we will attend the church where our children will be happy." I was relieved that they valued and listened to this perspective.

This story is not unique; I know many similar cases. As parents, it is important to reflect on the question: "Am I pleased with this church? What about my children?" We should consider not only our own interests but also the needs and happiness of our children.

It is important to note that not all parents prioritize their own interests to the detriment of their children. Some parents are genuinely concerned about what benefits both them and their children.

I have encountered parents who are receptive to advice regarding their children and value the perspectives shared with them. Conversely, there are also parents who prefer to follow their own methods and may decline to consider outside guidance, often stating, "I want to raise my children in my own way." This diversity in parenting approaches highlights the varying philosophies and beliefs that influence how families navigate decisions affecting their children's well-being.

One day, I encountered a father and asked him, "Why have you been absent from church? I haven't seen you and your children." He explained, "We have changed churches but plan to return." Curious, I asked, "Why?" He replied, "My wife likes your church." I then inquired about his children's feelings, and he mentioned, "The children do not like the church we are currently attending, but who listens to them? They are under us; they have to listen to their mother and father."

I responded, "I believe it's important to listen to your children as well." I added, "When you switch churches frequently, you may be depriving your children of a sense of stability, which can lead to confusion." The father acknowledged this, saying, "You are right, Wongel; to my surprise, my 7-year-old son is puzzled by our changing churches and has asked, 'Why do you take me from one church to another?'" I advised him, "We should settle down; otherwise, we risk raising unstable children. It would be best to choose a church where your children feel comfortable and receive sound teachings. Consider making a sacrifice for their sake."

He took my advice to heart and implemented it soon after. I have had similar conversations with other parents, and many have accepted my guidance. I appreciate their willingness to listen.

The topic of church community can evoke a variety of perspectives and experiences. For many, a church community serves as an essential support system, providing a sense of belonging and a space for spiritual growth. It often offers opportunities for fellowship, volunteer work, and shared values among its members.

In some cases, families may feel strongly about their choice of church based on personal beliefs, doctrinal teachings, or community involvement. Parents may consider their children's feelings when choosing a church, recognizing the importance of a stable and nurturing environment for their spiritual development.

However, there are also instances where parents make decisions based primarily on their preferences, which can lead to discussions about the balance between parental authority and children's input. Ultimately, the dynamics within a church community can significantly influence family life and individual growth, with each family navigating their unique relationship with their faith and community.

The concern about the messages we send to our children is an important topic for many parents. It is crucial to consider how our words and actions influence their perceptions and relationships with others. Children are impressionable, and the way we speak about others can shape their understanding of love, kindness, and forgiveness.

When parents inadvertently encourage negative feelings towards others, it can create confusion and strain relationships that could otherwise be positive. In the example of the 7-year-old girl who was influenced by her mother's comments, it demonstrates how quickly a child can adopt a mindset that may not align with values of love and acceptance.

The scriptural reference from 2 Timothy 3:14-15 emphasizes the importance of teaching children foundational principles from a young age. Instilling qualities such as love, mercy, and forgiveness reflects the character of positive moral teachings, helping children grow into compassionate and understanding individuals. Encouraging children to forgive and to embrace kindness can foster healthier relationships and a more positive outlook on life.

In nurturing the next generation, it is essential for parents to reflect on the seeds they are sowing in their children's minds and to prioritize messages that promote unity, understanding, and love. By doing so, they can help cultivate a generation that values compassion and embraces others rather than fostering division.

Sowing Good Seeds in Children's Minds

Some parents can be concerned. The responses they give to their children regarding why they don't take them to the church they love can be surprising.

There was a 7-year-old girl who had a fondness for me. One day, we encountered each other at a birthday party, but she seemed distant. I asked her, "What is wrong? You didn't hug me." She replied, "I am okay." Her older brother, who was present, said, "My mother told her, 'Wongel does not love you; ignore her; do not talk to her.' That's why she is cold to you." This revelation was disheartening. It's troubling to see innocent minds influenced in such a manner. I have not yet discussed this with their mother, as the children expressed their fear of her and asked me not to bring it up.

As parents, it is important to avoid corrupting children's minds with negativity. We are accountable for the messages we impart to them. Instead of sowing seeds of discord, we should fill their hearts with love, allowing them to grow in joy and compassion.

2 Timothy 3:14-15 states, "But as for you, continue in what you have learned and have become convinced of, because you know those from whom you learned it, and how from infancy you have known the Holy Scriptures, which are able to make you wise for salvation through faith in Christ Jesus." Paul shared this message with his spiritual son, highlighting the importance of teaching foundational values. If Paul emphasized these teachings to his own followers, how much more important is it for us to educate our children about the nature of love, mercy, and humility found in Jesus Christ instead of negativity? If someone offends you, such as Wongel, forgive her, for forgiveness exemplifies the nature of Christ. We should strive to walk in love.

Teaching Children Empathy and Understanding

Teaching children empathy and understanding is essential for fostering healthy relationships and promoting social harmony. Here are some strategies that can be effective in nurturing these qualities:

1. Model Empathy: Children learn a lot by observing the behaviors of adults. Demonstrating empathy in your interactions with others helps children understand its importance. Share feelings openly and show compassion in various situations.

2. Encourage Perspective-Taking: Help children consider situations from others' viewpoints. Discuss different feelings and reactions, asking questions like, "How do you think they felt?" This can promote a deeper understanding of emotions.

3. Read Together: Reading stories that highlight diverse experiences and emotions allows children to engage with characters and situations. Discuss the characters' feelings and decisions to help cultivate empathy.

I remember when I was a little girl, there was a lady named Aside who read us a book every night. Whenever she found the time, she would share a story with us. My favorites were

"Beauty and the Beast" and "Pinocchio." The way she narrated the books was highly engaging, and we became very attached to her. We loved it when she read to us.

Another favorite of mine was "Sleeping Beauty," along with "The Fox and the Hound" and "Snow White and the Seven Dwarfs." During my childhood, there weren't many books available, but the stories she read to us ignited a love for reading. Our time together made us cherish books, and it was evident how significant they are for young children.

4. Practice Active Listening: Teach children to listen to others and respond appropriately. Encourage them to ask questions and show interest in others' experiences, which can enhance their understanding and connection with peers.

5. Promote Kindness and Helping Behaviors: Encourage children to engage in acts of kindness, whether it's helping a friend or volunteering in the community. These experiences can reinforce the value of caring for others.

6. Discuss Emotions: Create a safe space for children to express their feelings. Discussing emotions—both their own and others'—can help children recognize and validate a range of feelings.

7. Use Role-Playing: Role-playing different scenarios can help children practice empathy in a safe environment. This interactive approach allows them to navigate complex social situations and develop their understanding.

8. Encourage Diverse Friendships: Supporting friendships with children from different backgrounds can enhance understanding and appreciation for diversity. It provides opportunities for children to experience varying perspectives.

9. Reflect on Experiences: After social interactions, encourage children to reflect on what went well and what could be improved. This reflection helps them learn from their experiences and develop greater emotional intelligence.

If children are raised in an environment that promotes negativity, they may later criticize their parents for not instilling positive values. Teaching harmful behaviors can lead to their normalization as children grow older.

However, exposure to messages about love and forgiveness—such as those found in religious texts—can create a disconnect where children feel their upbringing did not align with these teachings.

The Bible verse Psalms 8:2 states, "From the mouths of children and nursing babies you have ordained praise," suggesting that children are born with an inherent capacity for goodness and love. This innocence can be easily disrupted by exposure to negative influences.

In settings like Sunday school, children may experience minor conflicts but typically resolve them quickly and return to friendship. Adult intervention in these disputes can sometimes lead to children developing grudges, as parents might instruct them not to associate with certain peers. As a result, children may express that they have been told not to play with someone, which can create sadness and conflict within their friendships.

This situation raises questions about the messages we communicate to children about relationships. By encouraging negative perceptions of others through parental guidance, we may inadvertently influence children to adopt vindictive behaviors rather than fostering their natural tendency for reconciliation and kindness.

If children are raised in an environment that promotes negativity, they may later criticize their parents for not instilling positive values. Teaching harmful behaviors can lead to their normalization as children grow older. However, exposure to messages about love and forgiveness—such as those found in religious texts—can create a disconnect where children feel their upbringing did not align with these teachings.

The Bible verse Psalms 8:2 states, "From the mouths of children and nursing babies you have ordained praise," suggesting that children are born with an inherent capacity for goodness and love. This innocence can be easily disrupted by exposure to negative influences.

In settings like Sunday school, children may experience minor conflicts but typically resolve them quickly and return to friendship. Adult intervention in these disputes can sometimes lead to children developing grudges, as parents might instruct them not to associate with certain peers. As a result, children may express that they have been told not to play with someone, which can create sadness and conflict within their friendships.

This situation raises questions about the messages we communicate to children about relationships. By encouraging negative perceptions of others through parental guidance, we may inadvertently influence children to adopt vindictive behaviors rather than fostering their natural tendency for reconciliation and kindness.

It is important for children to express praise and positivity. In Matthew 21:15-16, we see an example of this: when the children cried out, "Hosanna to the Son of David," some adults became indignant and questioned Jesus about their words. Jesus affirmed them, stating, "Yes. Have you never read, 'Out of the mouths of children and nursing infants you have prepared praise for yourself'?"

Childhood should be a time for teaching children to love, praise, and sing to the Lord, rather than instilling negative feelings such as grudges, racism, or malice. If there are parents who encourage harmful attitudes, it is essential to recognize the innocence of children. We should allow them to grow in that innocence. As children mature, they will inevitably encounter the complexities and challenges of the world, including negativity and corruption.

By cultivating a mindset of love and positivity in children during their formative years and protecting their innocence, we can help them develop the resilience to navigate the hardships they may face in the future.

PositiveParenting

Positive parenting focuses on nurturing children in a supportive and encouraging environment, promoting values such as empathy, respect, and kindness. This approach emphasizes the importance of guiding children away from negative influences, such as grudges and hatred, and instead instilling a sense of compassion and understanding.

By prioritizing positive values, parents can help children develop healthy emotional responses and effective problem-solving skills. Engaging in open dialogue about feelings, conflicts, and the importance of forgiveness can foster resilience and promote a positive outlook on life.

Creating an environment where positive behaviors are modeled and reinforced can empower children to navigate social interactions with confidence and empathy. Ultimately, positive parenting aims to equip children with the tools they need to build healthy relationships and contribute constructively to their communities.

Mindful parenting

Mindful Parenting is an approach that encourages parents to be fully present and engaged with their children. It emphasizes awareness of both their own emotions and the emotions of their children, fostering a deeper connection and understanding within the parent-child relationship.

By practicing mindfulness, parents can develop a greater sensitivity to their children's needs, behaviors, and feelings.

This can lead to more thoughtful responses to challenges and conflicts rather than reactive ones. Mindful parenting encourages setting aside distractions to focus on quality time with children, promoting active listening, and encouraging open communication.

Additionally, this approach can help parents model emotional regulation and coping strategies, which children can then emulate in their own lives. Overall, mindful parenting aims to cultivate a nurturing atmosphere that supports emotional well-being and promotes healthy development for both parents and children.

Avoiding Judgmental Attitudes in Parenting

All children are unique individuals. Even siblings, whether brothers or sisters, exhibit different traits, preferences, and abilities. For instance, one child may excel academically, while another may struggle with schoolwork. One might spend hours playing and running around outdoors, while the other may find joy in quiet activities at home. Additionally, some children may quickly drift off to sleep, whereas others may take a long time to settle down. Preferences for environments can also vary: one child may thrive in a bustling, noisy atmosphere, while another might prefer a calm and tranquil setting. Furthermore, personalities can

297

differ significantly; one child may be naturally bashful, while another may be outgoing and bold.

Given these variations, it is important for parents to approach their children and others with an understanding of their specific behaviors and needs. The uniqueness of each child should be celebrated rather than compared against their siblings or peers.

Many parents within our community may have inadvertently made mistakes in their child-rearing approaches. For example, I remember my own experiences growing up. While many parents would praise their children for their achievements, my mother often did not extend the same encouragement to me. Instead, she would say things like, "If your children are intelligent, they should tutor Wongel," insinuating that I was not performing well academically. This led other children to laugh at me, making me feel isolated.

In our neighborhood, and among my family and friends, it seemed that everyone excelled academically. I struggled to understand what was taught in school and did not have a strong interest in learning; I faced my own challenges.

Ultimately, it is crucial for parents to nurture each child's unique qualities and provide support tailored to their individual experiences. By fostering an environment free from judgment and comparison, we can help children feel valued for who they are, which, in turn, promotes healthier development and stronger familial relationships.

The topic of learning disabilities, such as ADHD and autism, is often met with varying attitudes within communities. It is crucial to recognize that these conditions are developmental disorders rather than illnesses, and they can manifest in ways that may require understanding and support rather than judgment.

In some cases, children may grow up in environments where their differences are downplayed or dismissed, leading to a lack of acknowledgment and potentially preventing them from seeking the help they may need. This can have long-term implications, as individuals may face challenges in various aspects of life as they grow older.

Conversely, there are parents who are aware of their children's unique challenges and strive to address them. It is important to foster a culture of support and empathy rather than judgment, as labeling children can lead to negative perceptions and feelings. Instead of comparing children, focusing on their individual strengths and areas where they might need assistance is fundamental to fostering a more inclusive and understanding community.

Celebrating children's achievements is natural, but it's equally important to acknowledge and support those who may face different challenges. Every child has their unique journey, and fostering an environment of acceptance and support can lead to better outcomes for all children, regardless of their developmental differences.

A husband expressed his disappointment regarding children raised in their community who pursue professions like electrician, plumber, dentist, hairdresser, or organizer, implying a lack of respect for these career paths. The wife contributed to the conversation by referencing a "disease" that she believes predominantly affects the white population, noting that children from their community often drop out of school citing learning disabilities or autism as reasons. She pointed out that such conditions were unfamiliar to her when she lived in Ethiopia and labeled them negatively.

As they continued to express their criticisms of other children's paths, I found myself increasingly frustrated by their views. When the wife asked how I would feel if my child wanted to become a plumber, I responded affirmatively, clarifying that I see no shame in that profession. I emphasized that attending university should not be the only acceptable pathway, as each child's circumstances and aspirations can differ significantly. It is unfair to judge those who choose different routes or to diminish their ambitions because they do not align with traditional expectations. Hearing such judgments repeatedly is disheartening, as it perpetuates negative stereotypes and undervalues the diverse paths that individuals may choose in life.

Parental Expectations

Parental expectations can significantly influence children's self-perception and choices. Many parents hope their children will achieve high academic success and pursue prestigious careers, often equating professional status with personal value. This can lead to pressure on children to conform to specific paths, sometimes at the expense of their own interests and aspirations.

While some parents emphasize the importance of higher education, others may recognize and support vocational training or alternative career paths. The impact of these expectations varies greatly among families. When parents express disappointment in certain career choices, such as trades or creative professions, it can create tension in the parent-child relationship.

Conversely, when parents celebrate their children's diverse aspirations, regardless of societal norms, it can foster a more supportive environment. Ultimately, a balanced approach that values individual interests and abilities, alongside parental guidance, may be most beneficial for a child's development and well-being. Promoting a variety of career options and respecting each child's unique path can lead to healthier self-esteem and personal satisfaction.

Once, in a coffee shop, I was sitting with a sister while enjoying our drinks when a charming girl entered with her friends. This sister recognized the girl, and they exchanged pleasantries before she introduced me. I remarked to the sister, "She is charming; she is beautiful." To my surprise, she responded with sadness, "What is the value of beauty? She was born and raised here;in canada her parents had high hopes for her, but she disappointed them by becoming a hairdresser. Her brother is a computer animator. Their parents had aspirations for both of them."

I rebuked the sister, saying, "How can you make such a judgment? Would you be content if I spoke about you in the same manner?" She replied, "I am a refugee; I wasn't born here. Yet I have earned a degree. If I had a daughter born here who wished to be a hairdresser, I might feel utterly despondent." I was taken aback. A few moments later, I said to her, "You are being judgmental." I continued, "How can you presume to know if this girl has dyslexia, ADHD, dyscalculia, dysgraphia, or other learning difficulties?" She responded, "These issues often affect a spoiled child; it is people like you who accept such problems and fail to push forward."

When I told her, "You and I are fundamentally different; I didn't realize you held these views," she remained unfazed. Sipping her coffee, she stated, "You are newly acquainted with me; my opinions do not change because of your displeasure. I am simply speaking the truth." At that moment, I reflected, "I cannot continue a friendship with someone who views the world in this way." Thus, I decided to end our friendship, even though I cared for her. I thought to myself, "She will likely judge me similarly someday." I parted from her amicably.

This conversation highlights the complexity of individual aspirations and societal expectations, particularly within different cultural contexts. The sister's perspective reflects a strong belief in achievement and the pressures that come with high expectations from one's family, especially in immigrant or refugee situations. Her reaction to the girl becoming a hairdresser suggests that she views success through a specific lens shaped by her experiences and background.

On the other hand, your response emphasizes the import-ance of understanding individual circumstances, including potential learning disabilities, and recognizing that personal fulfillment can take many forms beyond traditional success metrics.

The decision to end the friendship speaks to a critical realization about compatibility in values and attitudes. It illustrates how differing viewpoints on success and judgment can create tension in relationships. Ultimately, it's important for individuals to seek connections with those who share similar values while also acknowledging that everyone has their unique journey and definition of success.

This experience might serve as a reminder of the diversity of perspectives in the world and the importance of empathy in understanding others' choices.

Understanding the Situation They Are Enduring

A young woman shared with me, "My parents hoped I would attend university, but I am facing academic difficulties. A doctor has diagnosed me with Dyslexia, which affects my ability to recall letters and understand what I have read. I am receiving medical treatment and taking medication, yet my parents are hesitant to discuss this with others."

When my parents confided in two individuals about my situation, they received the advice, "Do not accept what the doctor has said; they often mislabel healthy children as having illnesses." My parents took this advice to heart, telling me, "You are healthy; there is nothing wrong with you. Just keep praying and studying." Despite my efforts and prayers, I continued to struggle. As my difficulties intensified, my teachers called my parents to the school to discuss my challenges with my studies. My mother, unwilling to accept this reality, broke down in tears at school, praying in front of me. She lamented, "How could this happen, Lord? What have I done to deserve this for my daughter? You gave me only one child, and after so much hardship, do you make her sick?"

The emotions I experienced in that moment are indescribable. In my despair, I contemplated suicide that very day, telling myself, "I will not be a burden to my parents." I ingested some prescribed medication along with other substances and lost consciousness. I am unsure of what transpired during that time, but I was rushed to the emergency room, where I remained for two days. Afterward, my parents were frightened by the situation and accepted me for who I am. They sought my forgiveness, and I resumed my medication and education. Ultimately, I completed grade 12 and became a Critical Care Nurse, earning more than my parents.

She continued, "I do not hold any judgment against my parents. However, when some people remarked that 'their daughter is sick,' I believe that instead of feeling anxious or bitter about my situation, they could have chosen to support and encourage me more firmly. If they had embraced a perspective of gratitude, saying, 'Lord, we thank you for blessing us with this beautiful and intelligent daughter; we trust that you will turn this situation into something positive,' it might have made a significant difference. I feel that with that kind of encouragement, I may not have faced such overwhelming temptations."

Solution
Parental support

Parental support plays a crucial role in a child's emotional and psychological well-being, particularly during challenging times. In this case, the daughter's experience demonstrates how the response of parents to difficult situations can significantly impact a child's self-esteem and resilience. By fostering an environment of encouragement and gratitude, parents can help children navigate academic challenges and health issues more effectively. Instead of expressing anxiety or doubt, framing the situation with positivity and support may have created a more supportive atmosphere, potentially mitigating feelings of inferiority or failure. This example illustrates the importance of constructive parental attitudes in a child's development and coping mechanisms.

Avoid Viewing Your Child as Exceptionally Superior to Others

Some parents tend to describe their children as if they were flawless while perceiving other children as inherently problematic. I have encountered parents who consistently highlight the virtues of their own children, yet often discuss the difficulties of others. They frequently praise their son, stating, "He is impeccable; he detests wrongdoing; he even covers his ears upon hearing a secular song; he has no knowledge of any secular music." However, the reality of the children does not always align with their parents' portrayals.

I have taken the opportunity to share observations about their children's behaviors, pointing out, "There is no secular song that the child, who is said to 'have no knowledge of any secular song,' is not familiar with. Although he is described as 'decent,' he physically assaults other children, uses foul language, and causes distress among his peers; his behavior cannot be characterized as anything but unruly."

Avoid Perceiving Your Child as Exceptionally Superior to Others

Some parents tend to describe their children as if they were perfect, often viewing other children as inherently troublesome. I have known parents who consistently extol the virtues of their own children while frequently discussing the issues faced by others. They often assert that their son is "flawless;" they claim he despises wrongdoing, even going so far as to cover his ears when he hears a secular song, insisting he has no knowledge of such music. However, the reality of their children's behavior can differ significantly from these claims.

I have observed that while these parents speak highly of their children, the truth tells a different story. I pointed out to them, "There is no secular song that the child, who is reportedly 'unfamiliar with secular music,' does not know. While he is described as 'decent,' his actions include bullying other children, using inappropriate language, and causing distress among his peers; his behavior is far from commendable."

They were taken aback. "Are you talking about another child?" they inquired. I responded, "I am referring to your child." The father quickly retorted, "My son is a decent boy; it could be that he's influenced by so-and-so's child. So-

and-so lives in a troubled neighborhood, surrounded by negative influences; he is the one who has taught our son to swear."

I replied, "It is unjust to label the other child as 'bad.' Such attitudes do not align with what is right, and before attributing blame to others, it is essential to understand your own child's behavior. When you hold other children responsible for your child's shortcomings, your child may learn to shift blame onto others as well. This habit fosters irresponsibility, and, ultimately, they may lay their failures at your doorstep."

The responsibility of parents is not to cast blame onto others for their child's misbehavior but to guide them in shouldering their own responsibilities. We must refrain from harming other children by accepting our own child's claims without scrutiny; it is unjust to shift the blame for our children's mistakes onto innocent peers. When children are caught in wrongdoing, they often assert, "I didn't do it; so-and-so did." They say this out of a desire to evade punishment and avoid disappointing their parents. In such moments, it is crucial for us not to accept everything our children say at face value, nor should we rush to criticize other children.

Addressing Misbehavior

As mentioned earlier, I serve as a Sunday school teacher. During my time in this role, I occasionally observe behaviors in children that are unexpected. One day, while teaching, a girl unexpectedly poked a boy in the ear with a pencil, prompting a startled reaction from me. The boy began to cry, and I promptly placed the girl in a designated discipline chair and instructed her to apologize to him. Since her parents were delayed in picking her up, I left for home without informing them of the incident.

Later that day, I received a call from her mother, who expressed her concerns. She said, "Our daughter tearfully recounted what occurred today. How could you have made her sit in the discipline chair in front of the other children? She is very upset, and on top of that, you shouted at her. Our daughter is quiet, peaceful, and shy; I'm not sure we should continue bringing her to your class, as she may not return."

In response, I explained, "Your child should not have poked the boy in the ear, which is why she was seated in the discipline chair. Additionally, she had previously hit another girl without justification, and I had already warned her about that behavior." The mother then insisted, "My daughter would never do that." I offered to facilitate a conversation with the boy, as well as other children who had witnessed the incident, to corroborate my account. I noted, "Her action occurred in front of the other children, which is why I addressed it in the same setting; however, it was not meant to be punitive but rather a learning opportunity."

The girl's mother responded, "I can hardly believe what happened, but I will speak with the boy's parents." She later called me again to say, "The boy's parents are very upset; they didn't even want to talk to me. His mother told me tearfully, 'If Wongel hadn't been there, my son could have been seriously hurt.' She expressed her sadness over the incident.

The mother continued, "I am surprised by my daughter's behavior; she doesn't act this way at home or at school; she is typically very well-mannered." As she began to cry, I reassured her, saying, "This doesn't mean your daughter isn't a decent person; she is still a child and can make mistakes. However, it's important for her to understand that there are consequences for her actions. If she doesn't learn this, she might repeat the same mistake. If you are opposed to me addressing your daughter's behavior when it occurs, you may choose not to bring her to my class. I need to ensure the safety and well-being of all the children, and it is essential to discuss misbehavior to prevent it from happening again in the future."

Ultimately, the girl's parents apologized to me for the situation.

Child behavior can often be influenced by a variety of factors, including environmental context, peer interactions, and developmental stages. It is not uncommon for children to exhibit unexpected or inappropriate behaviors, as they are still learning social norms and the consequences of their actions.

When addressing misbehavior, it is important to approach the situation with a focus on teaching rather than punishment. Providing a clear explanation of the behavior and its consequences helps children understand the impact of their actions. Open communication between parents, teachers, and the children involved is essential for fostering a supportive environment where issues can be discussed constructively.

In instances where a child exhibits problematic behavior, timely intervention and guidance can be beneficial. This approach not only encourages better choices in the future but also contributes to the overall development of social skills and emotional awareness.

The purpose of sharing my experiences is to emphasize the importance of refraining from criticizing other people's children and confronting teachers solely based on your child's perspective.

To prevent unnecessary conflict, it is essential to listen to others, in addition to your child. It's important to recognize that every situation often has multiple viewpoints. I share this to encourage reflection and to help you avoid repeating mistakes. It serves as a reminder not to view your children as flawless and others as troublesome.

Taking a balanced approach can help foster a more understanding and supportive environment for all children involved.

Once, I noticed a child swearing. He was unruly and rebellious, often insulting his teachers indiscriminately in the classroom. I had reached my limit. I called him over, and said, "From now on, I will not tolerate your bad behavior. If you choose to insult others starting tomorrow, you will face consequences. For the rest of the day, I want to hear you using only kind words." Several students he had insulted were visibly upset and in tears. I added, "Now, apologize to them and to us." He complied, offering an apology.

After all the students left, he remained behind and asked, "Can I talk to you?" I replied, "Yes." He then said, "Do you know why I act this way?" I answered, "No, I don't." He continued, "Nobody wants to play with me; it makes me feel hopeless. Nobody loves me." Tears streamed down his face. I asked, "What makes you think that?" He responded, "I don't know." I reassured him, "Melkam, I care about you," and I hugged him.

When his mother eventually arrived to pick him up after a long delay, we were still embracing, and he was crying. She had never witnessed him hugging someone or showing such emotion before. This child had been struggling with behavioral issues since he was three years old, diagnosed with Oppositional Defiant Disorder (ODD). Unfortunately, he had not received the necessary support because his mother had stated, "I will not seek help," as she had not accepted the diagnosis. As a result, his behavior continued to deteriorate.

When he reached the age of five, no one wanted to be his friend. He had been dismissed from daycare as early as three years old due to his tendency to insult and hit other children. By the time he was six, the school he attended had already issued him two warnings.

He experienced ostracism at such a young age. Exclusion can lead children to develop harmful behaviors. His actions resulted in a lack of friendships; after all, who wants to be friends with someone who is constantly fighting? When his mother witnessed him hugging me and crying, she was taken aback and asked, "What happened?" I explained everything that had transpired.

His mother then shared her story. "I am a single mother raising him on my own. I've endured a lot before giving birth to this child. Whether you believe it or not, I had three miscarriages. When my husband realized I might not have children, he lost hope and left me.

After he left, I discovered I was pregnant. I told my husband joyfully, but his response saddened me. When I said, 'I'm pregnant; come and see me,' he replied, 'Since it's inevitable that you'll miscarry, I'm not coming; live your own life, and I'll live mine.' When I was nine months pregnant, I asked him to come and sign the birth certificate. He didn't believe it was true. After I gave birth, he signed the certificate but then withdrew from our lives. Since then, he has never visited our child; he only sends financial support. Out of love and a desire to cherish him, I have avoided punishing him, even when he insults me."

The mother reflected on her child's early behavior, recalling an incident when he threw a nursing bottle at her. This moment led her to indulge him, as she began to overlook his negative actions, including insults and hitting. As a result, he developed a pattern of behavior that went unchecked. Seeking to address his behavioral issues, she enrolled him in daycare.

However, once he started attending daycare, his disruptive behavior escalated, prompting teachers to suggest that he might have a behavioral problem. Instead of considering their feedback, she felt anger towards the teachers and opted to change daycare centers. Unfortunately, the new center also expelled him due to his behavior. When she attempted to discipline him afterward, her efforts were unsuccessful, and he entered school without the necessary support.

As he began school, complaints about his behavior continued to arise. Eventually, she decided to take him to a psychiatrist, who diagnosed him with severe autism. This realization was difficult for her to accept, and she initially resisted the diagnosis. She came to recognize that her indulgence and lack of discipline contributed to his challenges. Reflecting on her journey, she expressed regret for having labeled him as "rude," acknowledging the complexities of his situation and her role in it.

I suggested to the mother, "No matter what happens, he should show you respect. If you don't respond appropriately to his behavior, things will only get worse; he needs to stop insulting you." She nodded in agreement and expressed her sadness about her child's attitude towards both students and teachers. She apologized for any difficulties her son's behavior may have caused.

We shared a group hug, and I encouraged her to take him to a psychiatrist for further support. The mother demonstrated a commendable sense of accountability, stating, "This is my and my son's problem," rather than placing blame elsewhere. Over time, she has managed to build a successful life for herself, and her son is now attending school and receiving appropriate help. He has also made many friends.

Accountability refers to the willingness to accept responsibility for one's actions and their consequences. In the context of parenting, it involves recognizing how one's behavior and decisions can impact a child's development and behavior. Acknowledging accountability can lead to constructive changes aimed at addressing issues and improving situations. In this case, the mother took responsibility for her child's behavior and sought help, which ultimately resulted in positive outcomes for both her and her son.

Chapter Twenty Four

Avoid labeling other children as troublemakers

Some parents are quick to speak negatively about the children of others. For instance, they might label another child as "aggressive," "lazy," "indecent," or "rude." It would be wiser to observe and focus on children's behaviors rather than casting judgment on others' kids.

The child who clashed with yours likely had their reasons; they are not necessarily aggressive or mentally ill. It is possible that your child may have instigated the conflict. Just because your child came to you upset does not automatically imply their innocence. While some children do exhibit aggressive behaviors without provocation, it's crucial to recognize these instances and differentiate accordingly.

Merely listening to your child and always siding with them, regardless of the situation, can lead to greater harm than good. It's essential to consider both perspectives. By doing so, we can achieve a more balanced and effective approach. What I want to emphasize is that blindly supporting our child without question isn't always the best course of action. It may very well be that our child contributes to the conflict in one way or another. We often hear parents assert, "My child has been bullied; the troublemaker is so-and-so's child." It is more prudent to investigate what led to the situation instead of jumping to conclusions. In fact, declaring "So-and-so's child has bullied my child without justification" is not only misleading but can also have serious repercussions.

So, what are the characteristics of children who are often labeled as bullies? How can we identify them?

• They strive to dominate conversations.
• They often position themselves as victims.
• They may manipulate or deceive others.
• They engage in exclusionary behavior.
• They can be intimidating.

Being mindful of these traits can lead to a better understanding of the dynamics at play and foster healthier interactions among children.

If you notice children exhibiting behaviors such as those described, it is advisable to distance your child from them. It's important to reserve judgment when labeling a child as "a bully" without clear evidence of bullying behaviors. For instance, if our child is the one initiating physical contact and another child responds in self-defense, labeling the latter as a bully would be unjust.

Identifying female bullies can be particularly challenging. Typically, they may begin their bullying by ridiculing the way their victim dresses or mocking their accent. They often target various aspects of the victim's identity, forming groups to exclude the victim from social activities. They may also engage in behaviors such as hiding the victim's belongings.

If you observe these behaviors or if your child shares their experiences with you, it is important to take action and separate your child from those exhibiting such conduct. If bullying occurs in a school setting, it's crucial to report the situation to the homeroom teacher or the principal. If it happens in a church environment, informing the teacher or pastor is a responsible step to take. Addressing these issues proactively can help create a safer environment for all children involved.

Chapter Twenty Five

Avoid Judging Parents

It is common for people to quickly assume that a child's misbehavior is a direct reflection of their parents' actions or parenting style. Criticism often arises, with comments suggesting that the child's behavior is a result of inadequate guidance or poor upbringing. Phrases like, "He must have learned this from his parents," or "If they had set better boundaries, he would have listened," are frequently expressed in these situations.

When a child engages in activities such as substance abuse or theft, the instinctive reaction is often to place blame on the parents. However, this raises an important question: Do parents actively encourage their children to engage in harmful behaviors? It is rare to find a parent who openly instructs their child to take drugs or commit theft.

While it is true that some parents may struggle to effectively guide their children, it is also essential to recognize that not every instance of a child's wrongdoing is a reflection of parental failure. Historical examples, such as the sons of Eli in the Bible, illustrate that despite a parent's best efforts to guide and correct their children, those children may still choose to go down a different path. As noted in 1 Samuel 2:23-25, the sons did not heed their father's admonishments, highlighting the complexities of parental influence and individual choice.

It is important to approach situations of misbehavior with a balanced perspective, understanding that various factors contribute to a child's actions. While parenting plays a significant role in shaping behavior, it is not the sole factor at play. Recognizing this complexity can foster a more empathetic and constructive dialogue about child behavior and parenting.

A mother shared her experience of discovering sweets and toys in her young child's trolley, which led to a conversation with her husband. Initially, she found it hard to believe that her 3-year-old could be stealing, as he was too young to understand the concept. However, as her child grew older, his behavior evolved. At age 5, he began pocketing candies in supermarkets, and by age 7, he was lying about where he had gotten small toys.

Recognizing the seriousness of the situation, the mother decided to address her child's behavior directly. She explained to him the idea of theft and the consequences that come with it, including the concept of being put in prison.

He responded by asking about prison, prompting her to provide an explanation. After their conversation, he apologized.

This situation illustrates the complexities of child development and behavior. It highlights how serious conversations about ethics and right versus wrong can be essential in guiding children as they mature and navigate their understanding of social norms.

We thought he had given up since the day I spoke to him, but that hasn't been the case. I still find small items that he has taken. My husband and I are worried about this behavior; he has advised me, "Do not tell anyone." I reassured her, saying, "It's a mistake that you didn't explain these concepts to him when he was 3 and 5. If you had addressed it earlier, he might not have developed this habit.

If you're willing, I can talk to him." Moving forward, let's check everything before paying at the supermarket. If he tries to leave with any hidden items, either return them or pay for them." She agreed.

I then spoke with the child. I asked him, "Which of the sins sometimes trouble you? Choose three from the Ten Commandments. I ask this question of every child; you're not the only one. Most children pass the test by telling the truth, confessing their wrongdoings because the Lord loves us. We don't want to make the Lord, who cares for us, sad, do we? So, we must follow His commandments. By listening to Him, we uphold those commandments, right?"

He responded, "Yes." I then asked him, "Circle the sins that trouble you from these options." The choices included: do not kill; do not lie; do not covet; do not steal; honor your family; and others. He circled two: "do not lie" and "do not steal." I asked, "Why do you lie?" He replied, "My mother is often irritated with me; she cries, and my father gets angry. I lie because I don't want to see my mother upset."

I asked him, "Why do you think your mother and father get irritated?" He replied, "I do not know." I responded, "I don't believe they get irritated without a reason. What do you think it might be?" He said, "I think it is because I steal." I inquired, "Why do you steal?" He explained, "Whenever I ask my mother and father to buy me something, they say they don't have money and won't buy it; so I steal." I asked, "Are you aware that stealing is considered a sin?" He acknowledged, "I know it is a sin, but what can I do? I really like sweet foods, and they don't buy them for me."

I suggested, "Let's pray together. Ask the Lord to help you choose not to steal anymore and to ask for what you want instead. You can tell your parents too." He agreed, saying,

"Okay." While we were praying, he asked me not to tell his mother and father about our conversation. I replied, "Understood."

He then added, "Tell my mother and father to buy me what I want." I responded, "That's fine, but keep in mind that your parents may not be able to afford everything you desire. It's important to understand this. Also, remember that eating too many sweet foods can lead to tooth decay." He acknowledged this with a "yes."

I explained to him, "From now on, remember that the Lord sees you when you steal. Know that stealing also makes your mother and father sad; when they are sad because of you, you are violating another commandment." Before I could finish, he responded, "There is no commandment that says, 'Do not make your parents sad; you have not taught me that." I clarified, "You are violating the commandment to honor your parents." He seemed surprised and said, "You are right; the Lord will not love me, my parents will not love me, and all the people I know will not love me if I commit these sins."

I reassured him, "The Lord does not hate you; He hates your sins. Your parents will not hate you, but they do dislike your sins. If you choose to do wrong thinking your parents won't care, it will ultimately make them sad." His response was, "I will not make them sad again; I promise."

Later, while they were driving home, the child apologized to his parents in the car. His mother later shared that she was very pleased. He only stole once more after that incident, and even then, he immediately returned the item to his mother, saying, "I handed this to you because I do not want to violate the Lord's commandment."

I shared this story to illustrate that some parents may have children who develop poor habits during their childhood. It also serves as a reminder to refrain from judging parents without justification and to recognize that we can offer support to both parents and their children.

In general, we should avoid passing judgment on parents or individuals. Each child is unique, and it is important not to disparage someone else's child while elevating our own.

Rather than criticizing parents whose children have fallen into troubling behaviors, we should treat them with compassion and understanding. This is especially true for believers in the church, who should approach parents facing challenges with kindness and support.

Am I advocating for children or judging parents? How you perceive this speaks more to your own investments than to my intentions.

The church is not merely a gathering place; it is a sanctuary for outcasts, children, and parents who are hurting. When someone broken comes to the church, it is our responsibility to welcome that person with love. It is neither expected nor acceptable to exclude those with problems; that would be misguided.

In conclusion, it's important to remember that we should refrain from judging parents. Many parents face challenges that are beyond their control, and they often do not intend for their children to struggle with issues such as addiction, theft, or difficult behavior. Each child's circumstances are unique, and some behavioral issues can be particularly difficult for parents to manage. Rather than casting judgment, it is essential to approach these situations with understanding and empathy. Supporting parents in their efforts to help their children can make a positive difference for families in need.

Chapter Twenty Six

Word of Advice

To Children Under the Age of 12

When we allow our girls under the age of 12 to wear nail and hair extensions, lipstick, and similar enhancements, we unintentionally send a message that they should not accept themselves as they are. By adding these external elements to their appearance—elements that suggest they need alteration to be considered beautiful—we convey the idea that, "My daughter, you arc not beautiful as you are; if only you had longer hair, you would be beautiful." Although we may not express this sentiment in words, our actions speak volumes as these young girls grow up.

Introducing such embellishments can lead children to lose confidence in their own natural beauty. They may start to question their worth and compare themselves to others, resulting in lowered self-esteem. Children raised in this manner often find it challenging to accept themselves and may struggle with feelings of inadequacy. Such children might also experience frustration or anger when they see peers who conform to their ideals of beauty.

Conversely, when children are encouraged to appreciate their inherent beauty, they learn to praise God for the uniqueness and loveliness He has instilled in them. This appreciation fosters happiness and self-confidence. By nurturing their self-acceptance, we empower our children to grow into individuals who celebrate who they are.

One day, I encountered a sister in the Lord who had attached a hair extension to her 7-year-old daughter's hair. Out of concern, I expressed my disapproval, saying, "How could you allow her to wear that?" She responded with a smile, "Your daughter has beautiful hair; you cannot judge children who don't." She added, "Just remember, she's not your child—she's mine, and it's not your concern." The little girl, who was completely unaware of her thin hair, was influenced by her mother's comments. "You should wear this hair extension because your hair is thin," the mother would say, routinely adding the extensions. As a result, the child became so accustomed to wearing them that she wouldn't leave the house without one. It's truly disheartening.

When my daughter turned 14, some of her friends began experimenting with makeup. One day, she approached me and asked, "What do you think about me starting to wear some makeup?" I replied, "Where do you plan to get the money for that?" I only had basic items like lipstick and eyeliner, which she was aware of. She pointed out, "Other parents are buying makeup for their children." I acknowledged her statement but firmly responded, "That may be true, but I am not going to buy any for you." After our conversation, I went to my bedroom, closed the door, and prayed, "Lord, please help my daughter not to bring up the topic of makeup again." Since then, she has not asked about it again.

It is beneficial to avoid introducing children to makeup and hair extensions at a young age. If they choose to use these products when they are older, that decision should be theirs; however, we should not be the ones to provide them with such items.

When we adorn children, whom the Lord created beautiful, with artificial enhancements, we risk fostering low self-esteem as they grow up. As they mature, they may come to criticize us, saying, "My mother used to apply lipstick and other makeup or attach hair extensions to my hair because she thought I wasn't beautiful."

I recall a situation in which a 6-year-old girl came to school with her hair dyed purple. Many parents expressed their frustration with her mother because numerous children began requesting similar hair colors. This led to upset among parents, with some strongly opposing the idea of dyeing their children's hair. Such incidents highlight the importance of allowing children to be children.

We should pray for the Lord's guidance over our children while fulfilling our responsibilities as parents. It is essential to commit their wellbeing to Him and encourage them not to focus on artificial enhancements at such a young age. Our role as parents is to support their development in a healthy way while trusting the Lord with what comes next.

To Parents,

I would like to share some advice that may be helpful based on my own experiences. These suggestions are not meant to address major issues but rather to encourage positive parenting practices that can benefit our children:

• Avoid Teaching Racism: It is crucial to foster an environment free from prejudice and discrimination. Teach children to embrace diversity and appreciate differences among people.

• Instill Respect for All: Encourage your children to respect everyone, regardless of their background, beliefs, or appearances. This foundational principle can enhance their relationships throughout life.

• Promote Kindness and Sympathy: Teach your children the importance of being kind, sympathetic, and good-hearted. These values can help them develop strong emotional connections with others.

• Encourage Volunteerism: Instilling the habit of helping others can be transformative. Urge your children to volunteer their time and effort to assist neighbors or those in need, fostering a sense of community and empathy.

• Avoid Comparisons: Help children focus on their own strengths and growth rather than comparing themselves to others. This can support their self-esteem and promote a positive self-image.

• Set Boundaries for Desires: It's important not to give in to every request just because children are upset or crying. Teaching them the value of patience and understanding limits is essential for their development.

• Promote Awareness of Others' Circumstances: Discuss with your children the realities faced by those less fortunate. Help them understand that some children may not have enough food, clothing, or access to education. This awareness can foster gratitude and compassion.

By sharing these thoughts, my hope is to inspire parents to nurture a supportive and empathetic upbringing for their children.

To Parents,

It is important to consider how we raise our children and the habits we instill in them. Some key points to keep in mind include:

• Avoid Spoiling Your Children: Children who are overly indulged may face difficulties as they grow up. Setting appropriate boundaries helps them develop resilience and responsibility.

• Teach Gratitude: Encourage your children to express gratitude by saying "Thank you" for both small and large gestures. This fosters appreciation and respect for others.

• Maintain Consistency in Discipline: When your children do wrong, it's crucial to stand firm and not give in. Consistency helps them learn accountability for their actions.

• Encourage Politeness: Reinforce the importance of saying "Please" when making requests. This simple act can foster respect and positive interactions.

• Assign Responsibilities: Give your children small tasks at home. This helps them develop a sense of contribution and work ethic.

• Model Positive Behavior: Avoid engaging in conflicts with others in front of your children. They learn from observing how we handle challenging situations.

• Manage Screen Time: Today's children and teenagers often spend considerable time on various electronic devices. Common devices include:

• Smartphones: Used for social media, messaging, gaming, and browsing.

• Tablets: Utilize educational apps, games, and streaming content.

• Laptops/Desktops: Used for schoolwork, online classes, gaming, and leisure activities.

• Gaming Consoles: Popular for gaming and social interaction through multiplayer features.
• Smart TVs: Provide access to streaming platforms for movies, shows, and videos.

• Wearable Devices: Smart watches can be used for notifications, fitness tracking, and communication.

Understanding the impact of these devices on your children's time and activities is essential for promoting a healthy balance between technology use and other important aspects of life, such as education and personal interactions.

Guidance for Parents

As you navigate the task of raising children, consider the following important aspects to help them develop into well-rounded individuals:

• Encourage Sharing: Children often struggle with sharing, as it goes against their instinct to hold on to what they consider theirs. Teaching them to share promotes empathy, cooperation, and social skills.

• Teach the Importance of Apologizing: Helping children learn to apologize fosters accountability and strengthens relationships. It encourages them to recognize when they've hurt someone and the importance of making amends.

• Respect Their Social Choices: It's important not to pressure your children into friendships with individuals they are uncomfortable with. Encourage them to choose friends based on mutual interest and respect.

• Communicate Mindfully: Be cautious about sharing personal information with your children. Discuss life matters only if they are relevant to their understanding or benefit. This helps maintain appropriate boundaries and ensures they feel secure.

Additionally, a key idea to remember is that laws and principles are integral to human society. Understanding rules and expectations can greatly benefit children. It helps them learn to navigate various situations, whether at home, with friends, or in school. Familiarity with family and societal norms equips them to make informed decisions as they grow.

Establishing Family Rules and the Balance of Love and Discipline

Creating a set of family rules can provide children with clear expectations and a framework for behavior. Here are some key rules to consider:

• Handle People and Property Respectfully: Encourage children to treat others and their belongings with care and consideration.

• Knock at Closed Doors Before Opening: This teaches respect for privacy and helps children understand boundaries.

• Tell the Truth: Honesty is fundamental and fosters trust within the family and in relationships outside the home.

• Keep Your Teeth and Body Clean: Promoting hygiene is important for health and self-esteem.

• Expressing Love with Boundaries: While it is crucial to show love and affection to children, it is equally important to establish boundaries and discipline. Excessive love without guidance can sometimes lead to challenges, such as difficulties with limits and understanding social norms.

Discipline does not equate to punishment; rather, it encompasses teaching children about responsibility, consequences, and respect for others. A lack of discipline may hinder a child's ability to develop self-regulation and navigate relationships effectively.

The objective is to foster well-rounded individuals who feel secure in their environment while also grasping the importance of accountability and empathy. Balancing love with appropriate boundaries is essential for healthy development. Parents often find that when love is expressed without limits, it can become challenging to enforce rules or correct behaviors, as they may fear causing emotional harm. Striking a balance ensures that children feel both loved and guided, equipping them for a successful transition into independence.

Establishing Family Rules and the Balance of Love and Discipline

Creating a set of family rules can provide children with clear expectations and a framework for behavior. Here are some key rules to consider:

• Handle People and Property Respectfully: Encourage children to treat others and their belongings with care and consideration.
• Knock at Closed Doors Before Opening: This teaches respect for privacy and helps children understand boundaries.

• Tell the Truth: Honesty is fundamental and fosters trust within the family and in relationships outside the home.

• Keep Your Teeth and Body Clean: Promoting hygiene is important for health and self-esteem.

• Expressing Love with Boundaries: While it is crucial to show love and affection to children, it is equally important to establish boundaries and discipline. Excessive love without guidance can sometimes lead to challenges, such as difficulties with limits and understanding social norms.

Discipline does not equate to punishment; rather, it encompasses teaching children about responsibility, consequences, and respect for others. A lack of discipline may hinder a child's ability to develop self-regulation and navigate relationships effectively.

The objective is to foster well-rounded individuals who feel secure in their environment while also grasping the importance of accountability and empathy. Balancing love with appropriate boundaries is essential for healthy development. Parents often find that when love is expressed without limits, it can become challenging to enforce rules or correct behaviors, as they may fear causing emotional harm. Striking a balance ensures that children feel both loved and guided, equipping them for a successful transition into independence.

Adapting Your Parenting Approach

When considering parenting strategies, it's important to understand that different styles can have varying impacts on children's development. Here are some key points to consider regarding the balance of love and discipline in parenting:

1. Emotional Security: Children who experience consistent love and support from their parents are more likely to develop a strong sense of emotional security. This foundation can contribute to positive self-esteem and confidence as they grow.

2. Boundaries and Expectations: Establishing clear boundaries and expectations is vital for children's growth. Discipline plays a crucial role in teaching children about consequences, helping them understand what constitutes acceptable behavior, and promoting self-regulation skills.

3. Balance of Love and Guidance: A parenting approach that integrates warmth and affection with appropriate discipline can help cultivate resilience and adaptability in children. Striking this balance enables children to learn how to face challenges and make responsible decisions, equipping them with necessary skills for navigating life's complexities.

In summary, adapting your parenting style to include both love and discipline can create a nurturing environment where children feel secure while also learning important life lessons.

Adapting Parenting Approaches for Optimal Child Development

When it comes to parenting, understanding the unique dynamics of your family and your child's individual needs is crucial. Here are several considerations to keep in mind:

1. Long-Term Outcomes: Research indicates that children who receive both love and appropriate discipline are more likely to develop strong social skills, emotional regulation, and a sense of responsibility. These attributes are essential for navigating relationships and challenges in adulthood.
2. Individual Differences: Every child is unique; therefore, what works for one child may not work for another. Parents may need to adapt their approaches based on their child's temperament, needs, and specific circumstances. Flexibility can enhance the effectiveness of parenting.

3. Balanced Parenting: Effective parenting often involves a combination of love, support, guidance, and discipline, allowing children to grow into well-adjusted individuals.

Each family can find its own balance that best suits their values and dynamics.

4. Practical Strategies: Attend Family Gatherings: Engaging in family gatherings can strengthen relationships and provide a sense of belonging for children.

5. Adjust Your Parenting: Be willing to modify your approach to better support your child's developing needs.

6. Set Limits: Establishing clear boundaries is essential for fostering discipline and understanding consequences.

7. Foster Independence: Encouraging children to make their own choices helps them develop decision-making skills and self-reliance.

8. Make Your Decisions Clear: Communicating your expectations and decisions transparently can help prevent misunderstandings and promote cooperation.

9. Risks of Spoiling: While it is natural to want to shower children with love and material rewards, excessive indulgence can lead to some negative consequences. For example, spoiled children may struggle with:

10. Entitlement: They may develop a sense of entitlement, expecting rewards without effort.

11. Difficulty Handling Failure: Excessive spoiling can hinder their ability to cope with disappointment and learn from mistakes.

Challenges in Relationships: They may face challenges in forming healthy relationships if they expect others to meet their needs without reciprocation.

In conclusion, successful parenting is about finding a personalized approach that blends affection, guidance, and reasonable discipline. By avoiding the pitfalls of excessive spoiling and embracing a balanced strategy, parents can help their children thrive.

The Potential Downsides of Spoiling Children

While providing love and support is essential in parenting, excessive spoiling—characterized by giving children too much without requiring any effort—can lead to several challenges. Here are some potential consequences:

1. Entitlement: Children who are frequently indulged may develop a sense of entitlement, believing they deserve certain privileges or rewards without having to earn them.

This can lead to unrealistic expectations in various aspects of their lives, including relationships.

. Lack of Resilience: Constantly shielding children from challenges or disappointments can hinder their ability to develop resilience. Facing setbacks is a crucial life skill, and children who are not allowed to experience failure may struggle to cope with difficulties as they grow older.

. Diminished Motivation: When children receive excessive rewards without effort, they might rely on external validation rather than cultivating intrinsic motivation. This can result in a lack of drive to set and achieve personal goals, potentially affecting their future success.

. Challenges in Social Relationships: Spoiled children may encounter difficulties in forming healthy peer relationships. They might struggle with important social skills, such as sharing, empathy, and cooperation, which are essential for developing and maintaining meaningful friendships.

In summary, while the intention behind spoiling may be rooted in love, it is important for parents to strike a balance that encourages children to appreciate their experiences, overcome challenges, and develop the skills needed for successful interactions and personal growth.

The Importance of Balanced Parenting and Its Impact on Child Development

While nurturing and caring for children is vital, excessive indulgence can lead to various challenges in their development. Here are additional potential consequences of spoiling children:

. Behavioral Issues: Children who are overly indulged may struggle with behavioral problems, as they often do not learn to respect boundaries or understand appropriate social behaviors. This lack of understanding can create challenges both at home and in school.

. Emotional Regulation: When children are shielded from disappointment, they may find it challenging to regulate their emotions. As they grow into adulthood, they might encounter difficulties coping with life's challenges and setbacks.

To promote healthy development and foster resilience, it is essential for parents to find a balance between love, support, and teaching responsibility. Here are some effective strategies for parents:

• Stay Involved: Maintain an active role in your child's life, showing interest in their activities, experiences, and feelings.

• Adapt Your Parenting: Be flexible in your approach, adjusting your parenting style to meet the needs of your child as they grow and change.

• Set Limits: Establish clear boundaries and expectations to help children understand what is acceptable behavior, promoting a sense of security.

• Foster Independence: Encourage children to take on age-appropriate responsibilities, helping them develop confidence and self-sufficiency.

• Explain Your Decisions: Communicate thoughtfully about parenting choices, helping children understand the reasons behind rules and limits.

Ultimately, a good parent—regardless of gender—takes an active interest in their children's well-being, aiming to create a nurturing environment that supports growth. By making time for children, boosting their self-confidence, and serving as positive role models, parents can foster well-rounded development and prepare their children for success in life.

A Love Letter
Wongel Gebeyehu

Chapter Twenty Seven

The Life We Should Have

Holiness

The Bible in 1 Peter 1:15 states, "But just as he who called you is holy, so be holy in all you do; for it is written: 'Be holy, because I am holy.'"

The Lord declares that He is holy and expects us to strive for holiness as well. While it may be challenging to live a holy life, it is important to remember that through His grace, all things are possible. To be holy means to be set apart for God, to separate ourselves from the ways of the world and to turn away from sin. The scriptures caution us against conforming to the patterns of this world (Romans 12:2). Instead, we are encouraged to be transformed by the renewing of our minds.

In our spiritual journey with God, committing ourselves to reading, meditating on the Word, and applying its teachings in our daily lives is an essential aspect of cultivating a holy attitude. When we earnestly pursue holiness, we naturally distance ourselves from sin and draw closer to Jesus Christ. Being in His presence transforms us; as we reflect His character, we become filled with meekness and humility.

Let us delve further into the concepts of meekness and humility and explore what the Bible reveals about them.

Meekness

The character of Jesus embodies meekness and humility. An important distinction to make is that biblical meekness should not be confused with weakness, fear, or a lack of strength and moral character. Instead, meekness represents an attitude of mind that stands in opposition to harshness and contention; it is expressed through gentleness and tenderness toward others.

Jesus exemplified meekness throughout His life, even as He spoke boldly, fully aware that His words could lead to torture and execution. Despite knowing that Judas would betray Him, He chose to share a meal with him, saying humbly and without anger, "What you are about to do, do quickly."

In our contemporary world, we often struggle to treat even those who are faithful, loving, and honorable towards us with fairness and respect. The idea of sharing a meal with someone we know is about to betray us seems unfathomable; we might even ignore such a person without justification. Today, there appears to be little meekness within the church. We frequently hear the notion that "If

you are meek, people will walk all over you." Consequently, I have witnessed many meek individuals transform
into bitter ones. When I ask them about this change, they
often respond, "Meekness does not pay off; if you are meek,
people will take advantage of you." Yet, the Bible
consistently encourages us to embrace meekness.

Meek individuals embody the character of Jesus, focusing
on the positive aspects of others and refraining from
harboring negative thoughts. Their actions are marked by
blessings and peace, reflecting the essence of Christ. Jesus
demonstrated this meekness in His interactions with those
who doubted or betrayed Him.

For instance, in John 20:27-28, we see Thomas expressing
doubt about Jesus' resurrection. Rather than expressing
annoyance or frustration, Jesus responded with compassion, inviting Thomas to reach out, saying, "Stop doubting
and believe." This gentle approach led to Thomas declaring,
"My Lord and my God" upon touching Jesus' wounds.

Additionally, Judas was not the only one to betray Jesus;
Peter also denied Him during His time of suffering. Despite
witnessing this, Jesus continued to embody meekness.
Today, we may encounter similar situations where friends
or acquaintances betray, suspect, or slander us. Regardless

of such challenges, embracing meekness remains important.

Humility

Humility is a term that is often misunderstood; many people equate it with weakness. However, being humble does not imply being weak. The Lord Jesus is the perfect example of extraordinary humility. Despite His divine status, He washed the feet of His disciples, demonstrating His humility. Please refer to John 13:4-10.

When we walk in humility, we may not always receive the respect we deserve; some may disregard us or even treat us with contempt. In John 8:50, Jesus reassures us, saying, "I am not seeking glory for myself."

I recall an experience with a sister in our church who seemed unwilling to greet me. I approached her with a humble spirit, but she did not reciprocate. She selectively avoided engaging with me, and when I greeted her, her response was minimal. Over time, she began to hide from me to avoid interaction altogether. Eventually, I chose to stop greeting her to prevent any discomfort for both of us. Although she has mocked my humility, I have not been hurt by her actions. It is surprising that, despite her service to the Lord, she displays contempt toward others, including myself. Nonetheless, we must continue to walk in humility as expected of us.

In the past, I might have reacted differently and ignored her entirely. However, I strive to embody humility because the teachings of Scripture encourage me to do so. Jesus maintained His humble disposition even in the face of false accusations and slander; from Him, we learn the importance of living a life marked by humility.

My father's favorite saying resonates deeply: "Humility is not fear; meekness is not weakness; but humility and meekness are certainly spiritual forces."

When we read the entirety of 1 Peter Chapter 3, verse 15 stands out in teaching us how to embody humility. This passage encourages Christians to take pride in their faith and to submit our concerns to the Lord with gentleness and reverence. We are not called to condemn those who are curious about our hope, nor to seek revenge, act conceitedly, or insult those who disagree with us. Instead, we are to display Christ-like meekness and humility in all our interactions. It is my daily prayer that the Lord will cultivate a spirit of meekness and humility within us.

Chapter Twenty Eight

Let Us Pray More Often

The Lord Jesus dedicated a significant part of His life to prayer, approaching it with a deep sense of purpose and burden (Mark 1:35; Luke 6:12).

Throughout His life, Jesus relied on prayer to navigate His trials. As we face our own challenges—be it trials, persecution, grief, despair, marital issues, or other struggles during our time in the flesh—we can find strength and solace through prayer. Just as prayer was an integral part of Jesus' everyday life, we too should cultivate a routine of entrusting every aspect of our lives to Him. By committing our concerns to His care and leaning on Him, we deepen our trust, which is nurtured through prayer.

Prayer should extend beyond the confines of church; it is vital to pray in our homes, in our cars, and wherever we may be. We should seek the Lord's presence consistently, in every situation and at all times—whether we are experiencing joy or sorrow.

My mother is deeply devoted to prayer. She prays when she returns home from work and even rises during the night to pray before starting her day again. I am continually amazed by her prayer life; her consistency is remarkable. She cannot go a single day or night without seeking the face of the Lord, committing everything to Him.

What I have learned from her is the value of prayer. I feel filled with joy as I share my thoughts and concerns with God, closing my door for a moment of solitude. It brings me happiness to approach the Lord with questions that exceed my understanding or to plead on behalf of others. I believe the Lord delights when we direct our gaze toward Him.

1 Thessalonians 5:17-18 states, "Pray continually, give thanks in all circumstances; for this is God's will for you in Christ Jesus." This passage clearly instructs us to pray without ceasing. Additionally, we are encouraged to pray for one another; James 5:16 reminds us, "Therefore confess your sins to each other and pray for each other so that you may be healed. The prayer of a righteous person is powerful and effective."

While praying alone is beneficial, praying with other believers is even more powerful. When one believer prays for another, it can provide significant encouragement. Jesus exemplified this by praying with His disciples and teaching them the importance of prayer throughout His life, as seen in Luke 23:46 and 5:16.

As Jesus prayed for others, we too should do the same. Ephesians 6:18 reminds us to "always keep on praying for all the Lord's people."

Philippians 4:6 encourages us: "The Lord is near. Do not be anxious about anything, but in every situation, by prayer and petition, with thanksgiving, present your requests to God."

A person who spends time in prayer radiates an uplifting presence. The words they speak carry goodness, and the joy of the Lord is evident in their demeanor. Such a character reflects God's nature, making them someone others are drawn to.

In these challenging times, it is God's will that we increase our prayers and include others in our petitions. May God pour His grace upon us and bless us abundantly with a life of prayer.

Chapter Twenty Nine

The Lord Who Works Through All

"But the Lord said to Samuel, 'Do not consider his appearance or his height, for I have rejected him. The Lord does not look at the things people look at. People look at the outward appearance, but the Lord looks at the heart.'" — 1 Samuel 16:7

Often, I observe individuals showing disdain for others based on superficial traits, especially after discovering that someone is uneducated or facing challenges. Phrases like "She is educated; she is beautiful; she should be a minister" and "He is educated" permeate discussions.

However, the Lord does not evaluate us based on our educational achievements; He examines our hearts. If God judge us by human standards, none of us would be worthy to serve Him. This is why the Lord often chooses to work through those who are marginalized and unexpected.

Take the apostle Peter, for instance. He possessed neither silver nor gold, but he had the authority of Jesus Christ. In Acts 3:5, we read, "Silver or gold I do not have, but what I do have I give you. In the name of Jesus Christ of Nazareth, walk." The story that unfolds after this declaration is remarkable.

Do not be surprised if you face disdain or persecution today. The apostle Paul and many believers throughout history endured numerous trials for their faith in Jesus, and the same happened to Jesus Himself. If you hold on to Jesus—seeing Him as your support, refuge, and guide—you will find hope even in the most challenging situations. He will lift you up when you stumble and fall.

The Word of God assures us: "God is mighty, but despises no one; He is mighty and firm in His purpose." — Job 36:5. Do not let the opinions of others disturb you. Instead, stand firm on the Word of God. He is the Lord who works through all individuals, regardless of their background—whether educated or uneducated, rich or poor, white or black—as He sees fit.

Chapter Thirty

Do Not Limit Yourself

"Do not limit yourself because others have limited you."

It is important to remember that when we encounter problems, it may be an opportunity for growth and overcoming challenges that God presents to us.

Let us reflect on the story of Esther. She came from a challenging background, lacking formal education and facing societal prejudices related to her race. Orphaned at a young age, she lived with her uncle Mordecai, who had high expectations for her despite their difficult circumstances. Her singular asset was her beauty, but even that did not confine her potential.

When a beauty contest was held in the citadel of Susa, many young women participated, undergoing extensive preparations. While the competition was intense, Esther stood out and gained favor with the king, exhibiting grace and confidence without succumbing to anxiety.

Esther, who was often overlooked due to her circumstances, not only found favor in the eyes of the king but also in the eyes of everyone around her. This demonstrates how divine assistance can lead to extraordinary outcomes. Her rise to queen was a testament to the power of God's favor in the face of limitations.

It is crucial to recognize that limitations do not define us. Many may view themselves as unworthy or incapable due to education, status, or appearance; however, one's worth is not determined by external factors. Just as God saw beyond Esther's external limitations, He sees the potential within each individual.

Those who judge based on appearances—whether it be education, wealth, beauty, or charisma—are overlooking the deeper qualities that matter. It is my hope that we can foster understanding and support among one another, choosing to build each other up rather than tear each other down.

Chapter Thirty One

Relying On the Lord

Throughout my life, I have encountered numerous hardships and adversities, often reflecting on how I managed to persevere through them. It is by the grace, power, and love of God that I have been able to navigate these challenges. Many Christians suggest that true faith should eliminate despair, labeling it as a sign of weakness or lost faith.

However, I can attest that there have been many moments when I felt overwhelmed and despaired, despite the presence of God's grace and word in my life. There were times when I found myself pleading with the Lord, reaching a point of darkness where I questioned my purpose. In those moments, I would cry out, "Lord, take me; if you do not, I am going to end my life."

Yet, during times of deep despair, it was the word of the Lord that breathed renewed hope into my spirit. Even in my bitterness and hopelessness, I received the message, "I will not die but live, and will proclaim what the Lord has done" (Psalms 118:17).

The reality of the Christian journey is that it is not always a continuous upwards trajectory. Moments of deep discouragement are part of the experience. I have learned that in such moments, turning to God in prayer, often through tears, is essential. As Billy Graham wisely said, "I have my moments of deep discouragement. I have to go to God ... and say, oh God forgive me or help me."

This chapter serves as a reminder that reliance on the Lord is crucial, especially during our low points, and that it is okay to experience despair. The key lies in recognizing it and seeking God's help to lift us back up.

Trials are an unavoidable part of life; they affect us all. In moments of difficulty, it is common to feel hopeless. However, regardless of how discouraging a situation may seem, it is important to rely on God and commit our challenges to Him. Reflecting on my own experiences, I recognize that had I given in to despair during my darkest moments, I would have missed the opportunity to help others facing similar struggles today.

When faced with hopelessness, it can be beneficial to remind ourselves to find stillness and acknowledge the presence of God in our lives. It's common for prayers to not be answered as swiftly as we hope, leading to feelings of abandonment or discouragement. It's essential to remember that God's timing differs from our own. Therefore, it's crucial not to resort to desperate measures during tough times. Trusting in God, even when circumstances remain unchanged, is vital.

God encourages us to place our trust in Him wholeheartedly. In times of despair, we may be tempted to take matters into our own hands, but true strength lies in waiting patiently for God's guidance and timing. Maintaining this faith can provide the peace and hope needed to navigate life's challenges.

We often divert our attention from the Lord and depend on our own knowledge and understanding. However, the Word of God instructs us to have complete reliance on Him. It emphasizes the importance of trusting in God wholeheartedly. Do not feel the need to know everything on your own; instead, place your trust in God's power in all aspects of your life. After all, it is God who watches over you in His unique way.

Chapter Thirty Two

My Life Lessons

1. Owe no one anything, except love.

2. Avoid comparing yourself to others.

3. Engage in activities that you enjoy.

4. Focus your heart on what is good and your mind on what is upright.

5. Remember that there is always someone who may excel beyond you.

6. Be quick to listen and slow to judge.

7. Steer clear of spreading rumors.

8. Strive to help others not only with your finances but also with your time, prayers, physical strength, and any resources available to you.

9. Let go of greed.

10 It is important to support the needy when you have both money and knowledge.

11 Treat others as you would like to be treated.

12 Do only what you are able; you cannot please everyone.

13 Do not look down on anyone.

14 Always remain open to learning from others.

15 Address your pride and strive for humility.

16 Do not be concerned about those who unjustly hate you and tarnish your reputation.

17 Speak positively about the good qualities of others whenever you can.

18 Avoid evil.

19 Focus on living your own life.

20 Trust in Jesus and allow Him to be your source of joy.

21 Ensure that God is a priority in all aspects of your life.

22 Be mindful of your time; avoid engaging in trivial matters, as time is valuable and irreplaceable.

23 Steer clear of individuals who only feign affection. Avoid individuals who do not have genuine feelings for you.

24 Don't expect anything from others.

24 Place your trust in the Lord, not in people.

25 Engage in what you enjoy.

26 Live a simple life and make time to relax.

27 Don't take pride in your knowledge, beauty, or wealth; these things are temporary.

28 Distance yourself from anything that disrupts your peace

29 Stay out of matters that do not concern you.

30 When you listen to a story, remember that there are two sides to every situation. Don't take sides; approach it with a neutral perspective.

31 What you sow, you will reap, whether good or bad."

32 Protect your thoughts from the influence of negativity

33 Don't make assumptions.

A Love Letter
Wongel Gebeyehu

- Be resolute: Throughout life, it's common to experience setbacks and challenges. What often helps is a determined mindset and support from a higher power. Remember that when you fall, you have the capacity to rise again. As noted in 1 Corinthians 16:13, standing firm is important.

- Never put off until tomorrow what you can do today: Whether it's household tasks or professional responsibilities, it's beneficial to complete what you can today rather than delaying. As mentioned in Matthew 6:34, it's wise not to worry about tomorrow.

- Set a goal: Having a goal in life can provide direction and purpose. While you may not always achieve your goals, striving for them is valuable. Many people pursue various aspirations, but some may not realize their dreams simply because they don't take the first steps. It's important to have goals, regardless of their size, and to actively work towards them without unnecessary delays.

- Seeking Guidance for Goals: It's common to feel uncertain about setting new goals. Desiring to align with what is meaningful to a higher purpose can guide you. Seeking clarity through prayer and

371

reflection on Scripture may help you discern areas where you can love and serve more effectively.

- Avoiding Judgment: It's crucial to refrain from judging others based on their choices or past actions. Understanding that everyone has their own circumstances and challenges can foster compassion. People can change, and it's important to recognize and accept who they are now rather than focusing on their past.

- Focusing on Your Unique Path: Comparing yourself to others can lead to feelings of despair, as each person has their own divine plan. Rather than measuring your journey against others, it's helpful to celebrate your own journey and what you have been given. By shifting your focus to God's provisions and keeping your mind on Him, you can maintain peace and work towards the goals intended for you. Remember, true fulfillment and direction come from Christ, and allowing Him to take the lead can guide you effectively.

- Insecurity and Comparison: It's widely recognized that feelings of insecurity often stem from comparing our own lives—particularly the struggles we face—to the curated highlights of others' lives.

This tendency can lead to the belief that everyone else is doing better, when in reality, everyone deals with their own fears and challenges. Understanding that you are only seeing a portion of someone's life can help to mitigate the urge to compare.

-   Importance of Communication: Assumptions can lead to misunderstandings and conflicts within communities. It's common to see people engage in disputes based on what they think rather than seeking clarity. Instead, fostering open communication by asking questions and expressing desires can be crucial in preventing drama and fostering better relationships. This principle, as noted by Don Miguel Ruiz, emphasizes that clear communication can indeed transform interactions and, by extension, lives.

-   Choosing a Path of Joy: Living a life grounded in love, kindness, and positivity can lead to greater joy. Letting go of negativity, such as wickedness, envy, and hatred, aligns with the wisdom found in Proverbs 10:12, which suggests that love can heal and mend conflicts.

- The Impact of Love and Kindness: Acts of love and kindness create a ripple effect; they not only bless the receiver but also enrich the giver. This sentiment resonates with the idea that spreading love can uplift those around you and contribute to a more positive environment.

Walk in Life

Walk through life, and you will experience genuine joy. Eliminate wickedness, envy, and hatred. Remember, "Hatred stirs up conflict; but love covers over all wrongs." — Proverbs 10:12.

Love and kindness are never squandered; they always make a significant impact. They bless both the giver and the recipient. As Barbara De Angelis wisely said, "Spread love everywhere you go. Let no one ever come to you without leaving happier." — Mother Teresa.

Conclusion

This is a love letter to you, drawn from my own experiences. I have learned much from my relationship with God, for life is indeed a school. I have shared with you the ups and downs I've encountered, without holding anything back. Nothing comes from me; everything is from Him, through Him, and for Him. There is none like God. I continually thank Him for adding years to my life and for granting me the opportunity to share the truths I have learned through my experiences and the teachings of God. Blessed be His holy name forever and ever!

The Importance of Encouraging Hiking

I fondly remember hiking with my grandfather, my aunt, and her husband, as well as with my cousins during my childhood in Ethiopia. At that time, I didn't particularly enjoy hiking. My grandfather would lead us along challenging trails, regaling us with fascinating stories that made the experience enjoyable. Those moments were truly our hiking adventures.

The paths we traversed were often difficult, but reaching the summit of the mountain brought a sense of triumph. My grandfather would always pray at the top and encourage us to pray as well. However, more often than not, we would rush to find a large tree for shade to protect ourselves from the sun. Despite our distractions, there was something empowering about taking a moment to connect with ourselves and with God—free from the distractions of phones and gadgets.

Hiking not only allows for personal reflection, but it also helps to rejuvenate the spirit. My friends and I often find that when we're feeling stressed, rather than sitting down over coffee to discuss our problems, we choose to go hiking instead. It serves as a fantastic form of exercise, allowing us to appreciate the beauty of nature. Although scaling a mountain can be challenging, reaching the top brings a profound sense of accomplishment.

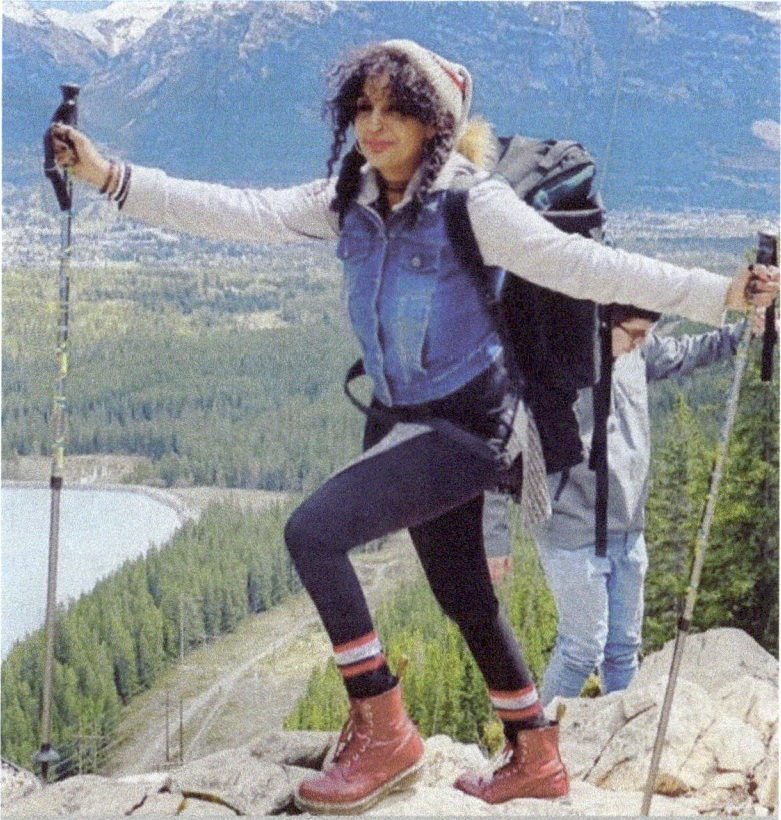

Life, much like hiking, presents its own set of challenges. It can throw obstacles our way, but with patience and perseverance, we can overcome them. Climbing to the summit requires effort, but the satisfaction of achieving our goals is worth it. Life is difficult; however, it's important to remember that we can reach our "mountains" if we keep striving toward them.

This is why I have a passion for hiking. As I navigate those winding trails, sometimes encountering bears or cougars that spark a bit of fear, I'm reminded of the parallels in life. No matter the challenges we face, if we remain determined, we can reach the top of the mountain.

Why I Like Hiking

Hiking offers a unique opportunity to connect with nature and escape the distractions of daily life. It allows for physical exercise and the chance to enjoy fresh air, which can be refreshing and rejuvenating. The experience of reaching the summit of a mountain or exploring a new trail can provide a sense of accomplishment and fulfillment. Additionally, hiking often fosters a sense of mindfulness and reflection, as it allows time for personal contemplation without the interruptions of technology. Overall, hiking combines physical activity, connection to nature, and moments of introspection, which makes it a valuable and enjoyable experience for many people.

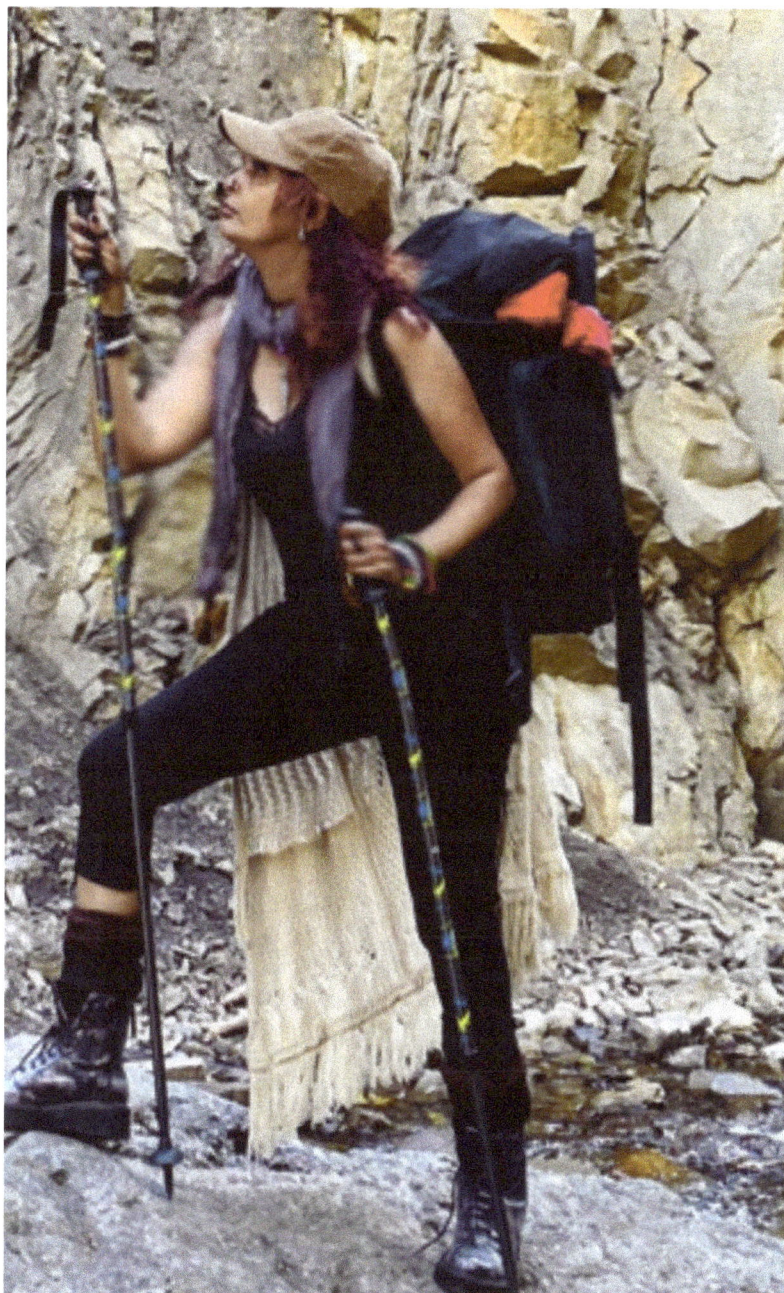

379

BENEFIT OF HIKING

1. Conncction with Nature: Hiking offers the opportunity to immerse oneself in the beauty of the natural world, fostering a deeper appreciation for the environment.

2. Physical Exercise: It is a great way to stay active and improve physical fitness, promoting overall health and well-being.

3. Mental Clarity: Spending time outdoors can provide a sense of peace and mental clarity, allowing for reflection and relaxation away from daily stressors.

4. Sense of Accomplishment: Reaching the summit of a trail or completing a challenging hike instills a sense of achievement and boosts confidence.

5. Social Interaction: Hiking can be a shared experience with friends and family, promoting bonding and creating lasting memories.

6. Mindfulness: It encourages a mindful approach to life, as hikers are often more aware of their surroundings and in tune with their thoughts.

7. Adventure: Hiking is inherently adventurous, offering the thrill of exploring new trails and discovering hidden gems in nature.

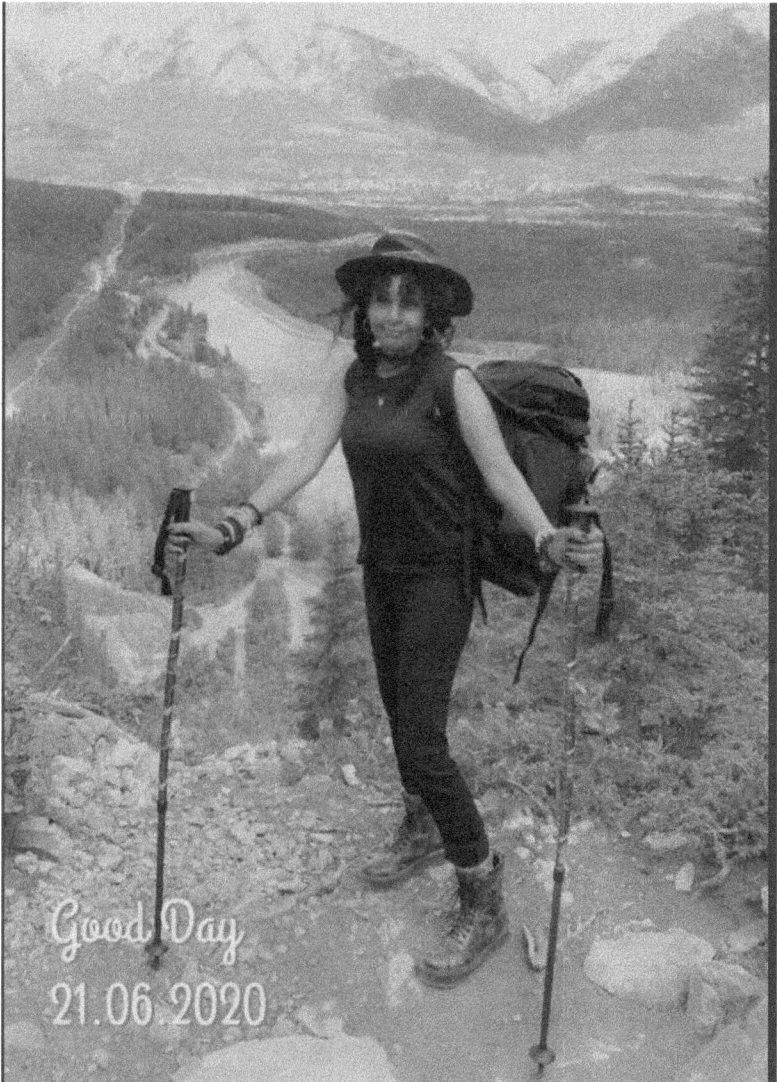

Hiking brings physical health benefits.

1. Cardiovascular Fitness: Hiking is an aerobic activity that can improve heart health, increase endurance, and enhance overall cardiovascular fitness.

2. Strengthening Muscles: It engages various muscle groups, particularly in the legs, core, and back, contributing to strength and stability.

3. Weight Management: Regular hiking can help burn calories, which can aid in weight management or loss.

"Hiking and climbing on top of mountains is what brings me the greatest joy in life," Wongel

My dream

My dream is for all your children to help a child in Ethiopia, Eritrea, or anywhere else to change their lives through support. By helping just one child, we can make a significant difference in the world. Give your children a purpose, so they understand that there is another child out there who struggles to survive. Encourage them to help—don't just tell them about it.

By assisting another child, we can raise a generation of passionate, loving, and kind individuals. If they can reach out to even one child in need, I promise you that we won't overlook those who deserve the opportunity to go to school, eat well, and have shoes. We are investing in the next generation and empowering them to succeed.

Your children will be happier because they will experience a sense of accomplishment from their acts of kindness. That's why I created the Kids to Kids program some time ago. Let's work together to make it a success and help those in need."

Bibliography

• Charles Stanley: When the Enemy Strikes, Blessings of Brokenness, How to Let God Solve Your Problems.
• Joel Osteen: Your Best Life Now, Becoming a Better You, You Are Stronger Than You Think.
• Joyce Meyer: Battlefield of the Mind, Change Your Words, Change Your Life, A Confident Woman, My Time with God.
• Oprah Winfrey: The Life Lessons and Rules for Success.
• Amy Robach: How I Let Go of Control, Hold onto Hope, and Found Joy in My Darkest Hours.
• Benny Hinn: Good Morning, Holy Spirit.
• Benny Hinn: The Mystery of the Anointing.
• Michelle Obama: Becoming.
• Toni Braxton: Unbreak My Heart.
• Hoda Kotb: Ten Years Later: Six People Who Faced Adversity and Transformed Their Lives.
• Tyra Banks: Modelland.
• Naomi Campbell: Swan.
• Viola Davis: Finding Me.
• Kerry Washington: Thicker Than Water: A Memoir.
• Miley Cyrus: Miles to Go.
• Hilary Duff: Elixir.
• Paris Hilton: The Memoir.
• Drew Barrymore: Wildflower.
• Prince Harry: Spare.

• Mindy Kaling: Is Everyone Hanging Out Without Me?.
• Priyanka Chopra Jonas: Unfinished.

• መጽሐፍ ቅዱስ: የ1954 ትርጉም. በኢትዮጵያ መጽሐፍ ቅዱስ ማኅበር የታተመ::
• መርዖን ወልደ ሐዋርያት (ፓስተር): ተግባራዊ ምክር. ርጥቦት አታሚዎች፤ አዲስ አበባ፤ 2013 ዓ.ም.
• ተከስተ ጌትነት (መጋቢ): እንደ ጻና ቀረ. ርጥቦት አታሚዎች፤ አዲስ አበባ፤ 2016 ዓ.ም.

The list continues with notable figures like Benny Hinn, Michelle Obama, Toni Braxton, Hoda Kotb, Viola Davis, Miley Cyrus, and many others, each contributing unique perspectives through their memoirs and reflections.

The selection of books that I 've read covers a wide range of topics, including spiritual guidance, personal challenges, and individual stories. This diverse array offers valuable insights and inspiration for readers interested in exploring various perspectives on the human experience. Each author shares their unique voice and journey, contributing to a deeper understanding of resilience, growth, and the complexities of life. Such a collection can serve as a beneficial resource for those seeking motivation or introspection regarding their own life experiences.

www.ingramcontent.com/pod-product-compliance
Lightning Source LLC
Chambersburg PA
CBHW050449270326
41927CB00009B/1672